"This is essential information to help persons with chronic fatigue syndrome find their way through the labyrinth of emotional and physical symptoms of this illness. Dr. Friedberg's book helps the patient sort through conflicting feelings and emotions and develop a model to improve overall well-being, comfort, and even productivity. The writing style is clear and designed to be readable by the person with CFIDS. The balance of this book is achieved by the experience of Dr. Friedberg as a CFIDS patient and as a trained counselor. It is this unique perspective that gives the book its value, and I would recommend it for both professionals and patients."

> —David S. Bell, M.D.,
> Harvard Medical School;
> author of *The Doctor's Guide*
> *to Chronic Fatigue Syndrome*

"This is an important book for people with chronic fatigue syndrome and their families, as well as the health professional who sees patients with this illness and wishes to understand them better."

> —Leonard A. Jason, Ph.D., CFS
> researcher and professor of
> psychology, DePaul University,
> author of ten books, including
> *Remote Control: Help for Families in*
> *a Television Age*

COPING *With* CHRONIC FATIGUE SYNDROME

Nine Things You *Can* Do

FRED FRIEDBERG, PH.D.

NEW HARBINGER PUBLICATIONS, INC.

Copyright © 1995 Fred Friedberg
New Harbinger Publications, Inc.
5674 Shattuck Avenue
Oakland, CA 94609

Cover design by Lightbourne Images copyright ©1995.
Text design by Tracy Marie Powell.

Distributed in U.S.A. primarily by Publishers Group West; in Canada by Raincoast Books; in Great Britain by Airlift Book Company, Ltd.; in South Africa by Real Books, Ltd.; in Australia by Boobook; in New Zealand by Tandem Press.

Library of Congress Catalog Card Number: 95-69480

ISBN 1-57224-019-9 paperback

First printing July, 1995, 7,000 copies
Second printing April, 1996, 3,000 copies

During the 18 months of writing this book, I received helpful feedback from many sources. I wish to thank Barbara Quick for a detailed and thorough review of the manuscript. With expert precision, she simplified technical language, clarified important issues, and added informative details to the text.

I also wish to thank Bill Zimmer, Pat Fennell, and Jennifer Shlaes for their thoughtful comments. Their time and effort is much appreciated. Finally, I thank Laura Plourde for her professional skills in preparing this manuscript.

Contents

What We Know About Chronic Fatigue Syndrome

The Short Version

- Chronic fatigue syndrome (CFS) often hits suddenly, bringing with it overwhelming fatigue and an array of debilitating symptoms. Following the onset of CFS, even ordinarily easy activities can bring on crushing exhaustion.

- Physicians and the research community have little insight into the causes or course of CFS, nor is there much useful information around concerning the treatment of symptoms. Perhaps because of this pervasive ignorance and sense of frustration at not having answers or aid, health-care providers are often lacking in respect, patience, and empathy in their attitude toward patients with CFS.

- Because research findings are inconclusive, most things about CFS are in dispute, including its very existence, its prevalence among the general population, and its relation to similar illnesses reported earlier in the medical literature.

It cannot be predicted if a case will be long- or short-term, whether emotional and behavioral factors play a role, or what precisely causes the illness.

- CFS is most likely an expression of physical, genetic, behavioral, and emotional factors. Biological factors include genetic and hereditary susceptibility, allergy history, possible immune system defects, and external pathogens. Psychological factors may include a history of depression and pre-illness stress. Social factors that may influence susceptibility may include an overcommitted lifestyle demanding high personal achievement and overresponsibility in taking care of others.

How It Starts

I have chronic fatigue syndrome. Perhaps I'm one of the lucky ones, because I'm able to continue my work as a clinical psychologist, and I've learned to tolerate the illness and create a rewarding life for myself despite an array of symptoms.

Fifteen years ago, I lived in New York City and enjoyed jogging twenty-five miles a week around the reservoir in Central Park. I can remember the exact date when my good health went to hell: April 30, 1980. I began to experience pressure-like headaches while running, followed by post-exercise fatigue that did not dissipate for several days. Being the typical overachieving CFS type, I continued to run, and tried to ignore these symptoms. However, they increased to the point where I could no longer do even a fraction of my weekly mileage. I stopped exercising for several weeks, until I felt back to normal again. Then I resumed exercising, walking instead of running—I thought I could tolerate such a mild version of my fitness program. But the headaches began again along with the fatigue. These symptoms persisted, and I began experiencing memory problems as well. I've come to the sad conclusion that I cannot do regular exercise or get into the good physical shape that I used to maintain; and I'm resigned to feeling abnormally tired most of the time.

For the past five years, I've taught coping skills and stress management workshops to other individuals with chronic fatigue syndrome. Through these group sessions, I've become well acquainted with about 100 people who are also afflicted with this disorder. Often, their symptoms began as suddenly as mine did, and the memory of the date of onset and the situation remains just as vividly etched in their minds.

One woman in a workshop I led remembered feeling a sudden, overwhelming fatigue while she was in the shower. Another patient of mine described a "crash" episode of fatigue, followed sometime later by symptoms of joint and muscle pain and lumps in the throat. I've heard such descriptions as, "It hit me like a brick," "I've never felt so debilitated in my life," and "Even getting up to brush my teeth was an effort." The sudden intrusion of CFS symptoms may be so overwhelming that you feel like you're dying.

CFS is a very stress-sensitive illness—and the stress you experience at the onset of the illness may represent the most wrenching experience in your life. The initial shock is related to severe debilitation, loss of income, uncertain diagnosis, rejection by physicians and significant others, and many other illness-connected concerns. An individual with early CFS may also experience a panoply of traumatizing emotions, including intense fear, confusion, and denial.

The worst symptoms for many people are their problems remembering, concentrating, or simply paying attention to their own thoughts in a logical manner. Many individuals with chronic fatigue syndrome also report a profound mental fogginess, which hinders carrying tasks through to completion, organizing their thoughts, and staying focused on their immediate goals. Even a simple distraction can derail their train of thought.

Some people with chronic fatigue syndrome suddenly develop panic attacks. These are brief episodes of terror or dread, accompanied by breathing difficulties, heart palpitations, a sense of impending doom, fears of going crazy, and a variety of other related symptoms.

People with CFS may reduce their working hours, or stop working entirely, due to crushing exhaustion. Activities that were easily tolerated in the past—such as physical exercise, housework, or even social conversation—now engender severe fatigue.

In the absence of a well-defined cause or treatment for the illness, few resources are available to CFS patients. Many physicians are openly skeptical of the existence of CFS, because no laboratory test is yet available to diagnose the illness. As a result, patients are often rejected or, at best, treated with an attitude of condescension. Even a sympathetic physician can offer only concern and palliative medications to treat symptoms. A support group may provide a feeling of shared coping; a psychotherapist, if he or she is knowledgeable about the illness, may be of some assistance.

Alternatively, a person with CFS may undertake a very time-consuming and expensive course of treatment from a nontraditional physician or other health practitioner. Often these people seeking help endure months or even years of mega-vitamin therapy, holistic remedies, IV vitamin infusions, and innumerable lab tests with little positive effect on their illness.

How This Book Can Help You

As both a clinical psychologist and a person afflicted with CFS, I've developed an arsenal of behavioral and emotional coping skills to deal with symptoms and maintain a high quality of life. In my coping skills workshops I've found that individuals with CFS can learn to alleviate depression, reduce stress, and modulate their debilitating CFS symptoms such as fatigue, headache, insomnia, and memory loss. In each chapter of this book, I discuss issues crucial to individuals with CFS from both a professional and personal perspective. This isn't an abstract, academic text: I know what you've been going through, and I think I have some strategies to help you cope with your symptoms.

The crux of personal control of CFS symptoms lies in the awareness of the subtle interactions between stress and symptoms: symptoms create stress, and stress, in turn, magnifies symptoms. A major stress can produce an easily recognized aggravation of fatigue or other CFS symptoms. But more often there is a gradual buildup of stress from physical and emotional sources that produces malaise, discouragement, and intensified CFS symptoms. This book will help you disentangle and minimize these negative interactions.

Coping With Chronic Fatigue Syndrome: Nine Things You Can Do will show you how to identify stress and diffuse its consequences through deep relaxation, cognitive coping skills, self-pacing, goal modification, avoidance of relapse triggers, and positive mood induction. I've also provided suggestions for designing healthy environments and improving your social support. These stress reduction and coping techniques are both easy to use and effective.

The material in this book represents an integration of my own personal, professional, and research experience with CFS. An acquaintance advised me to separate my personal and professional writing into two distinct books. Although I understand the logic of this suggestion, my perceptions of the illness have been shaped by my multiple roles of patient, clinician, and researcher. I believe that the interplay of these diverse viewpoints can advance our understanding of the illness.

A synthesis of personal and scientific perspectives underlies the concept of "coping strategies," a central feature of this book.

The value of this approach is illustrated in the text by the findings of empirical studies, the reports of patients, and my personal experience with the illness.

Finally, I don't want to leave the impression that good coping skills "cure" CFS, as some researchers have suggested. The illness *is* a debilitating medical condition that requires further research to determine causation, treatment, and cure. Fortunately, we have two national CFS organizations, statewide associations, local support groups, and three federally funded research centers dedicated to investigating the illness. The efforts of these organizations are only the beginning of what I hope will eventually herald the conquest of this baffling medical disorder.

I was encouraged recently by the findings presented at the 1994 International CFS conference sponsored by the American Association for Chronic Fatigue Syndrome in Ft. Lauderdale, Florida (Grissom 1994). Progress in understanding the illness was evident in several areas that I'll describe below.

CFS prevalence. The true prevalence of the disorder may be much higher than previously thought. The recognition of greater CFS prevalence will result in more pressure to increase research funding.

The persistence of CFS. Although many people improve over time, CFS *is* a chronic condition, not a self-limiting condition that resolves in some predictable manner.

Research findings on the brain and immune system. Further evidence was presented for a dysfunctional immune response in CFS, as well as abnormalities in brain function. Many speakers reported differences between CFS and control groups on physiologic measures. The next step is to demonstrate a consistent finding for CFS versus controls, and then to identify an abnormality that is *specific* to CFS. At this time, many CFS abnormalities are also found in other illnesses and in some healthy individuals as well.

The existence of Gulf War Syndrome. This condition is almost identical to CFS, and may afflict several thousand military personnel who were involved in the 1991 Gulf War. New research funding for this syndrome may yield a greater understanding of chronic fatigue syndrome.

For those of us with disabling symptoms, the research process is excruciatingly slow. I hope this book can offer useful skills while we await the research breakthroughs that will be needed to formulate an effective treatment and ultimate cure of CFS.

If you or someone close to you suffers from chronic fatigue syndrome, this book offers understanding and first-hand knowledge of strategies that have worked for me and others in regaining control of our lives, and navigating the rough waters of this illness. In deference to your limited energies, each chapter in this book is distilled to its main points ("Coping Strategies in a Nutshell").

You don't have to read the book sequentially. Scan the chapter previews and then read the sections that you think may be of most help to you right now. It may also make your life easier if your partner or significant other reads this book from cover to cover.

Defining CFS

In 1987 the Centers for Disease Control (CDC) published a case definition of CFS (Holmes et al. 1988). They defined the disease in terms of six months or more of persistent fatigue that severely restricted daily functioning, and the absence of any medical condition that could otherwise explain the fatigue. In addition, eight out of the following eleven minor symptoms had to be present:

- Generalized headaches

- Muscle pains

- Joint pains

- Mild fevers

- Sore throat

- Painful lymph nodes

- Muscle weakness

- Prolonged fatigue after exercise

- Cognitive problems such as memory loss or concentration deficits

- Sleep disturbance

- Abrupt onset of the illness

This initial CDC case definition became more controversial as new findings were published. Some researchers believed the definition to be too heavily weighted with psychological symptoms, so that it tended to include people with psychiatric disorders who did not necessarily have chronic fatigue syndrome. The definition failed to include other people with chronic fatigue syndrome who had relatively few symptoms. For instance, an individual with severe but fewer symptoms—such as unexplained, disabling fatigue, joint pains, and memory problems—would have been inappropriately excluded from a CFS diagnosis. One effect of excluding people with fewer symptoms was that studies of CFS prevalence may have substantially underestimated the number of individuals who suffered from the illness.

The new CDC case definition of chronic fatigue syndrome (Fukuda et al. 1994) responds to these concerns. CFS is now defined by

- *Unexplained persistent or relapsing fatigue of definite onset. The fatigue is not alleviated by rest, and results in substantial activity reductions from previous levels of work, study, social, or personal activities.*

- *Four out of eight additional symptoms must be present, including cognitive problems, sore throat, tender neck or axillary (armpit) lymph nodes, muscle pain, multi-joint pain, a new type of headache (often pressure-like), unrefreshing sleep, and debilitating fatigue following exercise.*

Clearly, the new case definition answers many of the criticisms made about the original diagnostic criteria. Rather than 8 out of 11 minor symptoms, the new definition requires only 4 out of 8. As a result, it's less likely that psychological disorders will be overrepresented, or true cases of CFS excluded. This new, less restrictive, definition, when used in epidemiologic studies, will lead to better estimates of prevalence of chronic fatigue syndrome. This is progress!

Prevalence of Chronic Fatigue Syndrome

Unfortunately, the underreporting of CFS by physicians may contribute to the perception that CFS is not an important public health issue. The 1993 physician-based CDC epidemiologic study (Gunn, Connell, and Randall 1993) found a relatively low prevalence rate: 2.0–7.3 cases of chronic fatigue syndrome per 100,000 individuals, or about 4–20,000 nationwide. By comparison, the estimated rate of coronary heart disease in the population is 7,000 per 100,000, and the prevalence of cancer cases is 3,230 per 100,000.

Dr. Leonard Jason (1993) of DePaul University offers several compelling reasons why the CDC-sponsored epidemiologic study may not reflect the actual prevalence of chronic fatigue syndrome:

- The skepticism of participating physicians about the existence of CFS may have resulted in its underdiagnosis.

- Many people experiencing unexplained fatigue probably turned to nontraditional medicine for relief of symptoms, and would therefore not be represented in the CDC survey.

- Low-income individuals who cannot afford ongoing physician-based care would also have been excluded from the CDC study. This latter group would be likely to include individuals with chronic fatigue syndrome who experienced major reductions in income due to their disability.

Of course, widespread skepticism among physicians about the legitimacy of CFS affects the reported prevalence of the illness. A recent survey conducted by a CFS support organization (Lewis and Wessely 1992) found that 57 percent of respondents reported that they had been treated badly or very badly by their doctors. Poor treatment may be partly a result of the medical community's attitudes toward fatigue in general. Among physicians—who are, after all, most responsive to symptoms they can address through medical intervention—fatigue has low priority compared to other signs or symptoms of illness. In contrast, people suffering from CFS usually rate fatigue as their primary symptom. Given the lack of effective treatments for persistent fatigue, it is not surprising that 75 percent of CFS patients, by one published estimate (Denz-Penhey and Mardoch 1993), have gone outside conventional Western medicine to find treatment for their illness. Given the unfortunate antagonism between CFS patients and the medical establishment, CFS epidemiological studies that rely on referrals from M.D.s will probably underestimate prevalence rates. An added problem is that individuals identified in these studies may not be representative of those people in the general population affected by chronic fatigue syndrome.

Dr. Jason has conducted his own community-based—rather than physician-based—epidemiologic study (Jason 1994) measuring the prevalence of CFS among a random sample of Chicago residents. He found an estimated 200 CFS cases per 100,000 individuals, a rate at least 20 times greater than that found in the CDC study.

A second community-based study conducted in the Pacific Northwest by Dr. Dedra Buchwald and colleagues confirmed Dr. Jason's findings. The Buchwald study estimated CFS prevalence to range from 98 to 267 per 100,000. This community-based study identified many high-functioning individuals with CFS who do not visit physicians for their illness—a subgroup that would have been entirely excluded from any physician-based study.

Why are these prevalence studies so important to people with chronic fatigue syndrome? Accurate prevalence estimates will substantiate the magnitude of the problem, and will mobilize public and private resources to address causation, treatment, and cure.

Getting at the Causes of Chronic Fatigue Syndrome

A Brief History of Illnesses Resembling CFS

Unexplained fatiguing illnesses have been described in the medical literature over the past 150 years. George Beard, a nineteenth century neurologist, coined the term *neurasthenia* (meaning loss of nerve strength) as a diagnostic label for a variety of symptoms quite similar to modern day chronic fatigue syndrome, including incapacitating exhaustion, marked reduction in activity level, joint pain, muscle weakness, and headache symptoms. Inability to work, impaired social relationships, and reduced recreational activity were all characteristic of neurasthenia. Cognitive complaints—such as forgetfulness, confusion, and an inability to concentrate—were also common.

Are neurasthenia and CFS the same illness? Despite the similarities, this question cannot be answered definitively. Not enough is known about either condition. However, one major difference between CFS and neurasthenia is the societal attitude toward these illnesses. Nineteenth-century neurasthenia was an accepted medical diagnosis: patients' suffering was taken seriously. CFS is viewed with skepticism by physicians and the society in general. The patient's ability to cope with the illness is strongly influenced by these cultural attitudes.

Over the past 60 years, numerous epidemic outbreaks of mysterious flu-like illnesses have occurred in communal settings, such as hospitals and army barracks. More recently, there were epidemics recorded in two small American towns, and among the members of a symphony orchestra. The prominent symptoms common to all of these clustered outbreaks included fatigue, headache, low-grade fever, sore throat, muscular aches and pains, depression, and cognitive complaints. Unlike individual, isolated instances of CFS, many (but not all) of these clustered occurrences of unexplained fatiguing illness recovered within a few months. However, most patients in the recent outbreaks in northern Nevada and upstate New York have *not* recovered.

Although the existence of these CFS-like illnesses shows that unexplained, debilitating fatigue is not a new phenomenon, little is known about their causes that might help us understand CFS.

What Predicts a Long-Term Case of CFS?

It has been suggested that pre-illness levels of stress and psychiatric disorder may predict who develops a long-term case of

CFS—although there is little evidence to support this viewpoint. One study found that a strong belief in physical causes of the illness predicted diminished chances for recovery three years after initial medical evaluation. What does this result mean? It could be interpreted to signify that a belief in physical causes prevents the CFS sufferer from addressing the underlying psychological causes. Alternatively, it can be argued with equal plausibility that those individuals in the study *accurately* believed their illness to have a strong biological component.

Another hypothesis is that poor coping skills maintain illness-related immune systems. However, a recent study of long-term CFS (Friedberg et al. 1994) failed to show any difference in coping skills between patients who were improving versus those who were worsening. I am not suggesting that good coping doesn't help, only that the relationship, if any, between coping abilities and illness progression has not been established. We do know that coping skills *are* associated with positive emotions and can improve functioning.

A Biopsychosocial Model of CFS

Twentieth-century Western medicine has endorsed a mind/ body dichotomy to describe illness. A disease is either psychological or physical. The categories are distinct and non-overlapping. Psychological disorders are trivialized as self-induced, self-maintained, and therefore amenable to self-cure. Physical ailments, on the other hand, are deemed "real," and command the respect and attention of physicians. Many people believe that an individual must have a recognized disease in order to be considered ill at all. And yet, in 50–70 percent of medical consultations, physicians cannot find a diagnosis to fit the patient's symptoms. CFS is hardly unique in this respect!

Fortunately, Western medical and psychological researchers have begun to more broadly define the concepts of illness and disease. The important interplay between mental and physical processes in chronic illness—long recognized by other cultures—can no longer be ignored by our society. The complete separation of mind and body is a cultural invention that runs counter to the latest medical research. Whereas heart disease and cancer were until recently believed to be solely "physical diseases," it is now well recognized that psychological and behavioral factors contribute to the severity and progression of these, and perhaps all, chronic conditions. Diet, activity level, and physical and psychological stress may all be important risk factors in heart disease, cancer, and diabetes—the major causes of death in the United States.

Rather than being purely of physical or psychological origin, chronic fatigue syndrome is most likely an expression of physical, genetic, behavioral, and emotional factors. I favor a "biopsychosocial model" to describe the illness, which acknowledges the complex and multifaceted nature of CFS (Ware 1993; Fennell, in press). Biological factors include genetic and hereditary susceptibility, allergy history, possible immune system defects, and external viral invaders (or other pathogens). Psychological factors that may be of influence include a history of depression and pre-illness stress. Such a history doesn't in any way compromise the reality of CFS. It only helps to explain how behavior and biology can interact to predispose an individual to a given illness. Social factors that may influence susceptibility may include an overcommitted lifestyle demanding high personal achievement and overresponsibility in taking care of others. If sustained over long periods of time, such behavior can produce chronic physical exhaustion.

CFS probably has several interacting causes that have to be defined for each individual. The contributions of biological, social, and psychological factors may be different for everyone.

Table 1 shows how individuals with CFS rate 11 possible causes of their illness in order of perceived importance.

Research on the Possible Causes of CFS

The precise causes of CFS are unknown. The sudden onset of flu-like symptoms in many cases, followed by persistent illness and fatigue, suggests a viral factor. However, analyses of blood samples from individuals with CFS have not consistently confirmed an association between any viral antibody, including Epstein-Barr virus, and chronic fatigue syndrome. Some researchers believe that CFS may be triggered by more than one viral agent and/or organic factors, such as immune dysfunction.

The investigation of immune function in CFS has yielded mixed results. Several controlled studies have found consistently impaired function of the natural killer cells which defend the body against tumor growth and viral infection. However, other measures of immune dysfunction have not been replicated. For instance, initial reports of elevated cytokine levels in the blood of CFS patients (cytokines are chemical messengers of the immune system that cause CFS-like symptoms) were not confirmed in the majority of patients in subsequent studies. These conflicting results may arise because CFS may have multiple causes that vary from one research sample to another.

Sleep disorders—including sleep apnea, hypersomnia, shaky leg syndrome, and narcolepsy—have been identified in a majority of CFS research subjects. Medical treatment of these sleep disorders can sometimes reduce CFS symptoms, but it does not eliminate them. It seems that sleep disorders contribute to debilitation in CFS; however, they are not the primary cause of the illness.

Recent studies of brain function in CFS have shown abnormalities that may be important to understanding the illness. A study of the hypothalamic-pituitary-adrenal axis in CFS patients (Demitrack et al. 1991) has shown deficits in cortisol, a stress-related adrenal hormone. Lowered cortisol has been linked to lethargy and fatigue. In contrast, clinical depression is related to abnormally high levels of cortisol. This study was the first to biologically differentiate CFS and depression. In a brain imaging study based on SPECT scan analysis (Schwartz et al. 1994), the findings suggested the presence of impaired blood flow in the temporal lobes of CFS subjects compared to depressed subjects and healthy adult controls. Impaired blood flow in the brain may have implications for understanding the cognitive deficits associated with CFS.

Two important milestones must be attained before we can pin down the causes of chronic fatigue syndrome:

- To be considered definitive, a research finding must clearly distinguish CFS from controls, and be replicated in several studies

- A biological marker must be *specific* to CFS and not occur in other disorders or in healthy individuals

---

Table 1. How 292 Individuals With CFS Rate Possible Causes of Their Illness

Perceived Cause	Respondents (%)
1. Immune/viral factors	90
2. Persistent stress	65
3. Genetic/hereditary factors	43
4. Toxic exposure	43
5. Allergies	37
6. Emotional trauma	37
7. Physical trauma	28
8. Diet	26
9. Vaccination/immunization	16
10. Consequences of pregnancy	9
11. Birth control pills/estrogen supplements	8

Friedberg et al. 1994.

Allergy, Immune Dysfunction, and CFS

Perhaps the medical condition most common among people with CFS is a history of allergy. With up to 85 percent of CFS subjects reporting a history of allergies, it's surprising that little research has addressed this issue directly. Dr. Stephen Straus and his colleagues have proposed that immune dysfunction, manifested as chronic overactivation of the immune system, produces the chronic flu-like symptoms associated with CFS, viral infections, allergies, and some psychiatric disorders. For as yet unknown reasons, the immune response in CFS may remain elevated despite the absence of any identifiable disease-producing agent. Such immune activation mobilizes cytokines, the chemical messengers that produce CFS-like symptoms. Figure 1 presents a simplified diagram of an immune activation model.

A Brief Overview of Immune Function

The immune system is designed to fight off invasions by bacteria, viruses, parasites, and cancer. All components of the immune system are involved in a particular fight, but only some components excel in fighting viruses, say, as opposed to bacteria or cancer. Under ideal conditions, the immune system decides which type of invasion is going on, and mobilizes those parts of the system that excel in fighting a particular enemy.

According to Dr. Lucy Dechene, chronic immune activation occurs in CFS patients—especially those with a history of allergies—when an invasion by a particular bacterium or virus (called the *pathogen*) is received as if it were a parasite. This response is *not* the best one. Either the pathogen never leaves the immune system, or the immune system does get rid of the pathogen, but has trouble returning to standby status. To use an analogy, the Cold War ended in the late 1980s, but the peace dividend never materialized. Similarly, the immune system is fighting a war against a nonexistent enemy, or it is fighting an actual enemy with the wrong weapons. To continue the political analogy, we're fighting a Vietnam instead of a Kuwait.

At the same time that the immune system is revving up to repel invaders, it is simultaneously releasing chemicals to depress itself. Why? Because the immune system is trying to control the escalating process of killing invaders: an overactive immune system will destroy you. That is, it will attack friendly tissue—your

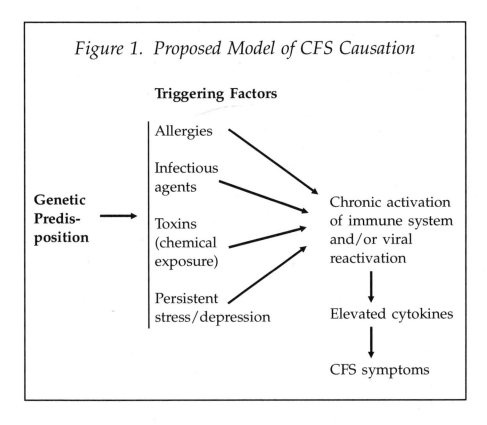

Figure 1. Proposed Model of CFS Causation

own—as well as true enemies. Like a peacetime army, the immune system needs to de-escalate its activity when the war is over.

To eventually depress immune functioning, histamine, cortisol, and other chemicals are released when the immune system is still actively fighting an enemy. Under ideal conditions, the depressive effects of these chemicals are pretty much ignored at the height of the invasion; but, as fewer and fewer immune complexes (antibodies stuck to the invader) circulate, the depressive action of the chemicals begins to work. In CFS, however, the immune system remains activated for a battle it cannot win and the system begins to overfunction destructively.

A Multidimensional Approach to CFS

Dr. Dechene (1993) proposed that the combination of persistent infection and an immune system defect produces many different types of fatigue. Rather than use the single vague term "fatigue" that is consistently misinterpreted and misunderstood, there may be several types of fatigue: "normal" fatigue, "allergy" fatigue, "fever" fatigue, "muscle" fatigue, and so on. By normal fatigue, Dr. Dechene means the natural tiredness a healthy person feels after a hard, active day. Allergy fatigue refers to the physical sensations arising from a small increase in histamine in the body (experienced by sensitive persons). Symptoms may include a feeling of heaviness in the limbs, general slowness of the body, muscle weakness, and mental sluggishness. Fever fatigue refers to extreme sleepiness, lack of mental alertness, muscle pain, and headaches that many people with even a slight fever experience. Each type of fatigue has a suspected physical cause that can be documented through medical research.

I present Dr. Dechene's model because I believe that it reflects the complexity of chronic fatigue syndrome. Rather than looking for a single "smoking gun" that explains the illness, Dr. Dechene proposes a multidimensional approach based on a thorough review of the relevant medical literature.

Dr. Dechene, Marjorie McKenzie, Robert Fontanetta, and I (1994) have completed a survey of 285 individuals with CFS as a preliminary test of the Dechene proposal. Four distinct clusters of fatigue symptoms were identified in our study:

- CFS relapse symptoms

- CFS remission symptoms

- Post-exercise fatigue symptoms

- Allergy fatigue symptoms that may reflect allergic or allergy-related sensations

On a personal level, perhaps you can identify differences in the type of fatigue you experience after exercising (if you are able to exercise) and the type of fatigue you experience during a setback or relapse related to stress or a natural fluctuation in the illness. These different types of fatigue may have overlapping, but not identical, physical causes behind them.

The different types of fatigue almost certainly interact with each other, and may be difficult to separate experimentally. We hope that our initial success in confirming a fatigue typology will stimulate research to verify the relationship between symptoms and proposed physiological mechanisms. If such confirmations are made, then medical treatment interventions could be customized to address different sources of fatigue.

If you have suspected or confirmed allergies, you can help yourself by minimizing exposure to allergy-producing substances. See the section on designing a healthy home environment in Step 8. Management of your allergy may reduce symptoms of fatigue.

Multiple Chemical Sensitivities

Figure 1 suggests that chemical exposure may be a contributing factor in CFS, although I'm unaware of any study that attempts to link environmental chemicals to the illness. Dr. Iris Bell, an expert on chemical disorders, proposed that an initial high-level exposure to a toxic chemical such as auto exhaust or an industrial pollutant, may sensitize the limbic system of the brain, which is responsible for regulating emotions. The limbic system is especially vulnerable to sensitization, and it is involved in generating emotions such as anxiety and depression that are associated with multiple chemical sensitivities (MCS). This sensitization process means that subsequent low-level exposures to the original toxic chemicals, as well as to other toxic chemicals, may produce debilitating physical and emotional reactions (listed below).

MCS encompasses a broad range of chronic conditions and complaints whose triggers may be low levels of common indoor and outdoor environmental chemicals, such as pesticides and solvents. MCS symptoms can include fatigue, depression, anxiety, irritability, mental fogginess, memory problems, insomnia, attention deficit disorder, and migraine headaches. According to the sensitization model, new low-level exposures—or persistent chronic exposures to the offending chemicals—will produce an increased physiological reaction. In other words, the MCS symptoms will increase with repeated chemical exposures. Since it is pretty much impossible to completely purge your home, neighborhood, and work environments of low-level chemical exposures, symptoms are likely to worsen over time.

How is MCS related to chronic fatigue syndrome? Many people with chronic fatigue syndrome report that they are highly sensitive to alcohol and medications. Lower-than-normal doses of prescription drugs will often produce a strong physical or emotional reaction. Alcohol, which cross-reacts with such environmental chemicals as auto exhaust, cannot be tolerated at all by many individuals with chronic fatigue syndrome.

In our recent study of people with chronic fatigue, a large percentage of the sample reported feeling ill ("often" or "almost always") in response to a variety of chemical exposures including pesticides (60 percent), tobacco smoke (59 percent), car exhaust (58 percent), perfume/cologne (54 percent), drying paint (52 percent), cleaning agents (52 percent), new carpeting (49 percent), and natural gas (for example, from a gas stove) (34 percent). In contrast, fewer than 14 percent of the spouses or significant others related to these people reported feeling ill in reaction to any of these substances. Are chemical sensitivities a contributing factor to chronic fatigue syndrome? We hope that our initial results may stimulate research into the relationship of MCS to CFS and its implications for the management of symptoms.

The Loading Hypothesis: A Comprehensive View of CFS

The immune activation model of CFS described above assumes a disruption in the body's ability to defend and protect itself. Why does this occur? The loading hypothesis, proposed by Dr. Seraphina Corsello, a holistic physician practicing in New York City, suggests that an accumulation (load) of physical and emotional stressors will adversely affect vulnerable individuals. These assaults to the body will lead to "exhaustion" of biological defenses and illness formation. The illness-producing stressors include exposure to allergens, toxic chemicals in the air, food, and water, and emotional stress. The breakdown of the body's defensive mechanisms (resistance) allows the takeover by viruses, bacteria, or other infectious agents.

Dr. Corsello's model provides an interactive view of environmental and biological factors in CFS. Given the high prevalence of allergies, chemical sensitivities, and pre-illness stress in people with CFS, the loading hypothesis has a commonsense appeal that matches the experience of many CFS-affected individuals.

Do People With Chronic Fatigue Syndrome Get Better?

Many CFS research scientists have expressed the belief that the illness is a self-limiting condition lasting from two to five years. Unfortunately there is little data to support the case for a duration of any given length. I've seen individuals get better within two years, although it hasn't been clear *why* they got better. Physical symptoms—such as fatigue and muscle pain—would resolve first; cognitive symptoms, such as memory loss, take much longer to improve. It seems that many people experience their worst symptoms during the first year of illness. Again, it's difficult to generalize about such information. The studies just aren't there.

Our recent long-term study suggests five basic patterns of illness progression in CFS:

1. Gradual improvements in symptoms over time with relapses and remissions along the way

2. Gradual improvements with illness severity roughly constant

3. No relapses or significant changes in the illness

4. Gradual worsening over time with relapses and remissions

5. Gradual worsening without relapses and remissions

Those individuals reporting the most severe symptoms during the first year of their illness reported the most improvement over time.

Three independent studies (including Wilson et al. 1994) have conducted follow-ups of one-and-a-half to three years after their initial evaluation of CFS patients. Remarkably consistent findings were presented: 60-65 percent of patients reported slight to significant improvements, while 25–35 percent reported that they'd become sicker. Only 2–8 percent reported complete recovery within three years. In considering these findings, it's important to remember that we don't know what factors predict a long-term case of CFS—or recovery, for that matter. It's probably most productive to sustain the hope that you'll be in one of the 2–8 percent who recover, or even one of the 60–65 percent who improve. Bear in mind that the combined improving and recovery categories *do* represent the majority of cases.

How Do People With CFS Rate the Treatments They've Received?

Categorizing and rating the effectiveness of all the medical interventions and experimental therapies that have been used to treat CFS is beyond the scope of this book. I can, however, present the results of our survey of people with chronic fatigue syndrome, and how they rated a variety of therapies.

Table 2 includes a list of treatments for CFS rated by 325 patients, including both long- and short-term sufferers. This information was collected from an international survey of people with chronic fatigue syndrome (Friedberg et al. 1994). The treatment that garnered the best result (the three people who tried it all reported moderate to major improvements) was Ampligen, which is an immune system modulator. A controlled study of Ampligen (Strayer et al. 1994) on 92 severely disabled people with CFS confirmed the efficacy of the drug in ameliorating the symptoms and disabilities associated with CFS. Unfortunately, Ampligen is no longer being produced or marketed in the U.S.

An anti-allergy diet helped 32 percent of the 186 respondents who tried it, while an anti-yeast diet was beneficial to 27 percent of a sample of 183. Antidepressant medications were helpful to 28 percent of the 249 people who tried them, although a substantial 31 percent of the patients reported that antidepressants made them feel worse.

As Table 2 shows, some treatments aggravated symptoms in a significant number of subjects. The interventions most likely to

Table 2. Treatment Effectiveness Rated by Individuals With CFS

Sample Size*	Treatment Tried	Moderate-Major Improvements(%)	Felt Worse(%)
3	Ampligen	100	0
186	Anti-allergy diet	32	<1
249	Antidepressant medications	28	31
183	Anti-yeast diet	27	5
133	Stress reduction/ biofeedback	26	<1
114	IV vitamins/ injections	26	4
180	Physical therapy/massage	26	16
109	Acupuncture	25	10
60	Kutapressin	25	12
65	Macrobiotic diet	23	15
184	Psychotherapy	19	7
283	Vitamin/mineral/ amino acid therapy	18	5
127	Allergy shots	17	27
129	Homeopathy	16	12
112	Tagamet or other H2 blocker	16	13

Table 2—continued

Sample Size*	Treatment Tried	Moderate-Major Improvements(%)	Felt Worse(%)
80	Malic acid	16	14
76	Gammaglobulin	16	20
38	IV antibiotics	16	39
207	Anti-inflammatory drugs	14	16
81	Antiviral drugs	14	19
195	Oral antibiotics	14	36
55	Removal of amalgam fillings	13	9
55	Magnesium injections	13	11
184	Herbal remedies	13	15
161	Co-Enzyme Q10	11	13
10	Transfer factor	10	30
44	Nitroglycerin	9	25
26	Alpha/Beta Interferon	8	23
17	Chelation therapy	6	12

From Friedberg et al. (1994)

* Sample sizes equal to or greater than 25 yield more reliable results.

worsen symptoms were IV and oral antibiotics (36–39 percent), antidepressant medication (31 percent), and transfer factors (30 percent).

Each individual in this survey tried an average of 9.4 treatments from the 29 listed. One conclusion that can be drawn from the results of this survey is that many people suffering from CFS are willing to try any number of treatments if they hold any chance of alleviating their symptoms.

Step 1

Identify Stress Factors: The Achieving Personality in CFS

Coping Strategies in a Nutshell

- Recognize that the tendency to overdo is a common trait in CFS.

- Identify the differences between the symptoms of CFS and depression.

- Compare your CFS symptoms to the comprehensive symptom list in this chapter. Have all new or unusual symptoms checked out by a sympathetic, CFS-knowledgeable physician.

- Become aware of the ways in which stress may aggravate your fatigue.

- Become aware of the ways in which negative, hopeless thoughts may contribute to stress and fatigue.

Why People With CFS Fight So Hard

> Self-professed desires for productivity, high standards
> for personal performance, and the tendency to "do for
> others" converge as the driving force behind this
> whirlwind of activity. These are people who describe
> themselves as "workaholics," "type A personalities,"
> and "perfectionists"—who would "go all out,"
> continually pushing themselves, to "do more" and
> "do it better." At the same time they complain of
> "having a hard time saying no," of "trying too hard to
> help others," of "giving too much" and consequently,
> "having too little left over" for themselves. The result
> is an exhausting lifestyle brought on by "overdoing,
> overworking, overtrying to please everybody and just
> overeverything." (From a study of 50 people with
> chronic fatigue syndrome by Dr. Norma C. Ware, 1993)

Dr. Norma Ware, a Harvard anthropologist, conducted in-depth interviews with 50 people with CFS in 1993. What she found was a lifestyle of high achievement and expectation involving full-time work, family responsibilities, and caregiving to others. Were these individuals happy with their active lifestyles? Dr. Ware doesn't appear to have asked that question directly. Based on my knowledge, I would say that most of these people probably enjoyed their lifestyles but felt overextended. The burden of overwork is certainly not unique to people with CFS. Since 1950, the average work week has been increasing, while personal relaxation time has diminished.

Were these overworking people in the study setting themselves up for a chronic illness? This question can't be answered until we're able to pin down the causes of the illness. Certainly, overstress may be a contributing factor. When I compared individuals with CFS to healthy adults and depressives, the people with chronic fatigue syndrome reported a significantly higher level of stressful events in the year prior to the onset of their illness, compared to the healthy adults. However, the depressed group reported an even *higher* level of stressful events in the year before they got depressed than the CFS group. The science of health psychology is only beginning to explore the role of stressors in the development of CFS and other chronic illnesses. Had we all known that we were risking illness with our lifestyles, would we have modified our activity level? *Had* we known this, at least we would have had a choice.

Are CFS people in general overachievers? I've collected a sizable data base on the personality styles and behaviors of people with chronic fatigue syndrome. Prior to the onset of illness, these individuals were very active. They averaged three-and-a-half times per week of vigorous physical exercise such as jogging, bicycling, or swimming. They worked at their jobs an average of 45 hours per week and still had time for 15 hours of active recreational and social pursuits. Obviously, there was no allowance in their schedules for colds or flu, much less a chronic illness. For highly active people, CFS is especially devastating. When I analyzed the reductions in activity following the onset of the illness, 40 percent could no longer work, and 26 percent had to reduce their workload to part time, while only 34 percent were able to maintain their full-time schedule of work and recreation.

Interestingly, the notion that a lifestyle of excessive work can cause persistent illness is not new. I found the following description in a 1923 book called *Chronic Fatigue Intoxication*:

> It affects almost exclusively the ambitious, the spirited and the strong-willed who, from a sense of duty or born on by their enthusiasm, drive their bodies beyond the limit of physical safety and who, before they are aware, have hypersaturated their system with fatigue material. (Ochsner 1923)

Fatigue and Depression: Understanding the Differences

Chronic fatigue syndrome is often accompanied by a depression-like state. Depression is, in fact, listed in the original CDC definition of CFS as one of the features of the illness. Some symptoms of CFS are identical to those that plague people with depression, including sleep disturbances, fatiguing easily, having difficulty concentrating, and feeling slowed down. When I use a standard depression scale with CFS patients, I raise the cut-off point for clinical depression, because I know that their depression scores will be elevated due to CFS symptoms, whether or not they are clinically depressed. Your own experience with the illness may have taught you to distinguish between CFS fatigue and fatigue related to depression. If you are often depressed about the illness, fatigue may simply appear to be an overwhelming, unchangeable entity that you cannot control.

A major assault to your body through chronic illness or injury can increase your vulnerability both to stress and depression. People who have been in severe accidents may, for the first time in their lives, experience stress and anxiety symptoms such as headaches, stomach distress, palpitations, panic, and fatigue. Chronic fatigue syndrome may similarly compromise your body, making you more susceptible to stress, anxiety, and depression.

To distinguish between depression and CFS, it can be helpful to look at the symptoms of depression that involve thinking—the so-called cognitive symptoms. If you're preoccupied with thoughts of worthlessness, self-criticism, and even death or suicide, and you consciously feel depressed, then you may be experiencing clinical depression as well as the depression associated with chronic fatigue syndrome. A key element in clinical depression that differentiates it from other medical illnesses is the loss of feelings of enjoyment or pleasure, or the loss of motivation to do things that you usually enjoy. Take a few minutes to fill out the standard depression scale (called the Center for Epidemiologic Studies Depression Scale or CESD) below. Scores above 25 are suggestive of clinical depression.

If you are depressed about your illness, it's certainly understandable. CFS brings about sudden and unexpected changes—most of them unpleasant—in your lifestyle. Your depression does not negate the fact that you're ill, and it doesn't mean that you're nuts. And fortunately depression can be treated medically and psychologically. See Step 6 for easy-to-use coping techniques to deal with depression. If you're preoccupied with thoughts of suicide or are too depressed to get up and get dressed in the morning, you

Center for Epidemiologic Studies Depression Scale

Below are a number of statements about the way you might have felt or behaved during the past week. Please read each statement and determine how often it was true for you during the last seven days. Use the scale below to score your answers.

0—Rarely or none of the time (true for less than one day)
1—Some or a little of the time (true for 1 or 2 days)
2—Occasionally or a moderate amount of time (true for 3 or 4 days)
3—Most days or all of the time (true for 5-7 days)

During the past week   Score

1. I was bothered by things that usually don't bother me. .... ☐
2. I did not feel like eating. My appetite was poor. .... ☐
3. I felt that I could not shake off the blues even with   ☐
   help from my family or friends. ....
4. I felt that I was just as good as other people. .... ☐
5. I had trouble keeping my mind on what I was doing. .... ☐
6. I felt depressed. .... ☐
7. I felt that everything I did was an effort. .... ☐
8. I felt hopeful about the future. .... ☐
9. I thought my life had been a failure. .... ☐
10. I felt fearful. .... ☐
11. My sleep was restless. .... ☐
12. I was happy. .... ☐
13. I talked less than usual. .... ☐
14. I felt lonely. .... ☐
15. People were unfriendly. .... ☐
16. I enjoyed life. .... ☐
17. I had crying spells. .... ☐
18. I felt sad. .... ☐
19. I felt that people disliked me. .... ☐
20. I could not get "going." .... ☐

Scoring: Reverse your answers for questions 4, 8, 12, and 16. 0 becomes 3, 1 becomes 2, 2 becomes 1, and 3 becomes 0. Now add up the numerical answers for items 1-20.

Fatigue Severity Scale

Below are nine statements exploring the nature and severity of your fatigue symptoms. Please read each statement and circle a number from 1 to 7, showing where you would locate yourself on the scale. One indicates the least agreement, and seven indicates complete agreement with the statement as it applies to your experience during the past week.

During the past week, I found that	*Completely Disagree*					*Completely Agree*	
1. My motivation is lower when I am fatigued.	1	2	3	4	5	6	7
2. Exercise brings on my fatigue.	1	2	3	4	5	6	7
3. I am easily fatigued.	1	2	3	4	5	6	7
4. Fatigue interferes with my physical functioning.	1	2	3	4	5	6	7
5. Fatigue causes frequent problems for me.	1	2	3	4	5	6	7
6. My fatigue prevents sustained physical functioning.	1	2	3	4	5	6	7
7. Fatigue interferes with carrying out certain duties and responsibilities.	1	2	3	4	5	6	7
8. Fatigue is among my three most disabling symptoms.	1	2	3	4	5	6	7
9. Fatigue interferes with my work, family, or social life.	1	2	3	4	5	6	7

Scoring: Add up your numerical answers and divide by nine.

should definitely get help from a trained helping professional without delay. Talk to your family physician or a CFS-knowledgeable physician if you need a referral.

The Fatigue Severity Scale (FSS) is another useful tool for differentiating fatigue from clinical depression. Take a moment to complete the nine-question FSS that follows the CESD scale. Then add up your numerical answers and divide by nine. Scores on the Fatigue Severity Scale range from 1.0 to 7.0. Scores between 6.0 and 7.0 are indicative of severe, persistent fatigue. Healthy adults average about 3.0 on the FSS. Depressed individuals without CFS score about 4.5. But CFS individuals average about 6.5, a highly significant elevation over depressed subjects.

What Is CFS, What Is Something Else?

A 28-year-old woman whose illness began ten months prior to joining my stress management group expressed her frustration about worsening symptoms:

> I couldn't understand each new symptom as I became
> more and more ill. I really started wondering if it's
> real or what. Every time a new symptom comes on I
> always go through this. Am I crazy, am I nuts, am I
> exaggerating? And then I realize it's there.

There is a laundry list of unusual sensations associated with CFS. For instance, many people with CFS experience diffuse aches and pains, numbness, and tingling. It's very difficult for anyone—including an expert on chronic fatigue syndrome—to say whether a particular symptom is related to CFS or something else entirely. If you're used to generalized aches and pains, and you get a couple more of them, you may ask yourself, "Is this related to my CFS, or is it something else?" Many people would follow with the question, "Am I becoming a hypochondriac?" Other people may tell you—and you may even tell yourself—to just ignore the new symptoms. And your doctor may say that they're nothing to be concerned about.

You have to decide for yourself whether a new symptom is important enough to be examined, and then endure all the skepticism you're bound to get from physicians. You vacillate between, "It's really nothing," and "Maybe it *is* something I should have checked out." This frustrating dilemma probably accompanies any new symptom you get.

Consider the following suggestions to deal with new symptoms:

- Find a sympathetic physician through your local CFS association, support group, other people with CFS, or the directory of physicians distributed by the Chronic Fatigue and Immune Dysfunction Syndrome (CFIDS) Association of America, P.O. Box 220398, Charlotte, NC 28222-0398 (1-800-442-3437). The National Chronic Fatigue Syndrome and Fibromyalgia Association also has comprehensive information about the illness. Contact them at 352 Broadway, Suite 222, Kansas City, MO 64111, (816) 931-4777.

- Reassure yourself that physicians *can* diagnose life-threatening or other serious illnesses if present, even if they can't properly evaluate CFS.

- Consult the list of symptoms below in Table 3. If your new symptoms are on the list, they may well be CFS-related, even if you haven't heard about them before. But be sure to consult a physician and insist on a full examination if you suspect that your symptoms may be related to something else. Always err on the side of caution and consult a professional if a symptom seems to warrant evaluation.

The Fatigue-Stress Connection

CFS sensitizes your body to stressful life events. Stress that would have been tolerated easily in the past now seems to produce an emotional overreaction. Even thoughts can illicit a feeling of overstimulation. Stress may trigger more fatigue and fatigue may create more stress. It can become a negative cycle as Figure 2 illustrates.

Table 3. Frequency of Symptoms Reported by CFS Patients

Symptom	Frequency (*Often or Almost Always*)
Severe fatigue	84%
Prolonged fatigue after exercise	82%
Muscle aches	78%
Forgetfulness	72%
Difficulty concentrating	64%
Sensitivity to light	59%
Difficulty thinking	58%
Less fluid gait	57%
Painful extremities	55%
Joint pain	53%
Confusion	52%
Insomnia	51%
Loss of sexual desire	51%
Extreme irritability	45%
Headache	43%
Bumping into objects	41%
Fever	40%
Numbness	40%
Shortness of breath	39%
Loss of balance going up or down stairs	37%
Dizziness	36%
Blurred vision	36%
Painful lymph nodes	34%

Table 3.—Continued

Oversleeping	32%
Sore throat	32%
Easily distracted when reading	30%
Depression	28%
Nausea	24%
Objects appearing closer/ farther than they actually are	20%
Rashes	21%
Painful menstruation	16%
Difficulty swallowing	15%
Burning sensations	14%
Requiring an aid (e.g., a cane) to walk	10%
Amnesia	7%
Vomiting	3%

Based on study of 300 CFS individuals by Friedberg et al. (1994).

Physical exertion (a stressor) may produce an immediate surge of fatigue, yet the most debilitating symptom flareups often occur several hours or a day later.

One workshop participant explained,

My car broke down and I had to walk about a quarter mile to get to a phone. The walk didn't seem that bad at the time. The next morning when I woke up, I couldn't move my bones around—it was like they needed oiling. Getting up made me feel like an old cat. It got so bad that I couldn't even get out of bed. I had a lot of things planned to do and then I realized where the stress was coming from—I never would have thought that the quarter-mile walk the previous day would flatten me. Now that I've made the connection, I can pace myself and plan a little better.

Emotional stress may also be a clear-cut fatigue trigger for some people. If you are one of these individuals, you may immediately experience very severe fatigue when you get upset. Yet for others with CFS, the effect of emotional stress is more subtle: you may experience a gradual buildup of fatigue symptoms and eventually recognize that upsets often trigger these intensified symptoms.

Typically, your physical symptoms are a direct expression of CFS. However, when you're upset, some CFS symptoms may worsen. There is an interface between emotional stress and physical symptoms which may be difficult to sort out, because the fatigue symptoms, whatever their source, will meld together.

This fatigue-stress interaction may increase the severity of your symptoms. This is how it happens: there are certain problems that cannot be resolved in any obvious or immediate way. For in-

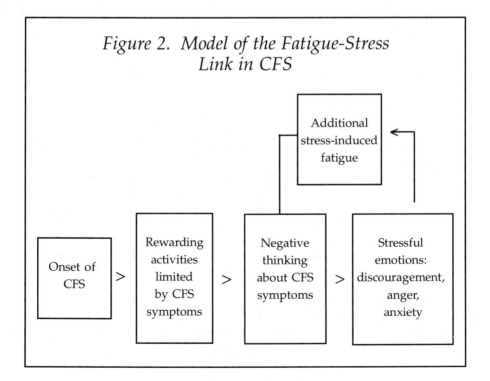

Figure 2. Model of the Fatigue-Stress Link in CFS

stance, many people with chronic fatigue syndrome carry a large burden of some kind, whether it be financial, vocational, marital, or family-related. When you think about these problems, a creeping feeling of discouragement—which serves as an added stress—may result.

Discouragement itself can be a very fatiguing experience. The fatigue from your discouragement interacts with the fatigue from your illness. The two types of fatigue bind together and intensify your symptoms. You're already fatigued because of the illness. Your discouragement from lifestyle changes and restrictions—and there are plenty of these—may lead you to feel hopelessly immobilized for a few hours, a few days, or even longer.

Of course, we all want to function at our highest level and not succumb to any form of discouragement. But symptoms and feelings may combine to magnify the burden of CFS. This is the result of emotional stress, and especially discouragement, adding to the burden of the fatigue. As you dwell on the fatigue and your other problems, discouragement intensifies.

One way to identify your fatigue-stress connections is to keep a daily log of symptom fluctuations. Table 4 contains a sample daily log with entries that illustrate the close connection between fatigue, stress, and depression. For this log, respondents use a 1-10 scale to express their fatigue level before and after a given event.

As the entries in the daily fatigue log show, any emotional stress, even a relatively minor one, can increase your feeling of fatigue. As you recognize how a series of minor events can cumulatively affect your fatigue symptoms and functioning, you can selectively practice stress reduction techniques, activity pacing, and the avoidance of unnecessary activities. These coping techniques will be explained in upcoming chapters.

Keeping a daily log for even a week will make you much more aware of specific stressors, and how they affect your mood and symptoms. Most importantly, the log will act as a starting point for changing negative interactions between stress and fatigue.

Make your own log in a notebook that you can easily carry with you. Then jot down stressful events as they occur. Make special note of the stressors that most increase your level of fatigue. These are the situations to avoid whenever possible. The following

Table 4. Daily Fatigue Log

Day and Time	Event	Emotional Reaction	Fatigue Level Before After 1 is lowest, 10 is highest	
Tues. 11:30 am	Argument with kids	Annoyance, frustration	5	6
Tues. 12:30 pm	Grocery shopping	Frustration	6	8
Wed. 8:00 pm	Social gathering	Worry, agitation, confusion	7	8.5
Fri. 1:00 pm	Meeting work deadline	Worry, pressure	4	6

chapters will suggest a number of different methods to deal with the routine stressors that are not easily handled when you have CFS.

Why Are Those CFS Patients So Angry?

> My doctor told me that all the tests were normal, and that I should see a psychiatrist to discuss early childhood experiences which undoubtedly are the reason why I'm "depressed" and chronically fatigued.

And people wonder why CFS patients are angry... One assignment I give to my CFS groups is to compose a list of ten things that make them mad. The initial reaction to that assignment is, "Are you sure you only want ten?" As high-achieving individuals, people with chronic fatigue syndrome are quick to blame themselves when they can't meet their own high standards. This self-anger and frustration can be an almost continuous reaction in early CFS when we doggedly attempt to maintain our pre-illness level of activity. We don't particularly spare ourselves from anger and blame. But plenty of hostility and frustration is also directed at judgmental physicians, unsupportive family and friends, and the divine being who may or may not have had some reason to make us ill.

We don't like to think of ourselves as angry people. Just give us back our health and we'll give up our anger. We have a right to anger. Perhaps anger gives us a temporary sense of power over an impossible situation. Perhaps it counteracts the helplessness we often feel. Perhaps the anger is a way to convince others that we are serious about the reality of our illness.

But anger costs us as well. It is a negative feeling that may deprive us of pleasant moments and enjoyable feelings. Anger seldom convinces anyone to be more receptive to our concerns. Often it backfires, creating more distance and less understanding.

Minimizing your anger may benefit your emotional and physical health. You can moderate your anger without compromising your determination to get the help you need, through lifestyle adjustments, medical intervention, CFS research, and a supportive network of people around you. Powerful methods to diffuse anger are described in Steps 3 and 6.

Adjustment to CFS: Denial or Preoccupation?

It's very important to articulate your thoughts and attitudes about CFS. Denying the illness or becoming preoccupied with it represent the extremes of coping behavior that we have all experienced. There is a healthier attitude in between these two extremes that you can define for yourself. With denial you may try to perform at 100 percent and pretend that everything is normal. If you have tried this, you know that it doesn't work for very long. If it did work, you wouldn't be shopping around for doctors, looking for support, or reading this book.

Preoccupation involves dwelling on the illness and shutting out the pleasant feelings that you still do have. You may start thinking over and over again, "I'm so sick, I'm so sick, and I can't stand this anymore." Such thoughts create depression and apathy, and can rob you of much potential enjoyment. If depression is already one of your symptoms, negative, hopeless thoughts will increase your depressed mood. If you are generally in a positive mood, but begin to become preoccupied with your illness, there may be a much more dramatic shift as your negative thoughts begin to predominate. It's hard to draw the line between healthy concern and maladaptive preoccupation with symptoms. Your daily log will help you make these distinctions. You can also use it to help you notice how much you dwell on symptoms. Specifically, write down your thoughts as well as your feelings in the daily log. For instance, if your thoughts are often focused on helplessness over your symptoms, then you have identified a target that can be constructively changed. Suggestions for changing negative thoughts may be found in Steps 3, 6, 7, and 9.

Step 2

Free Yourself From Expectations

Coping Strategies in a Nutshell

- If you don't have a confidant who will listen to you without judgment, find a support group or a therapist familiar with CFS issues. Call the CFIDS Association of America at 1-800-442-3437 for referrals. *Sharing your feelings will improve your ability to cope with your symptoms.*

- The most realistic goal you can set for yourself now is to perform at your full capacity within the context of waxing and waning symptoms. Holding yourself to your old expectations for achievement will worsen your symptoms and make you feel more miserable.

- Instead of simply enduring other people's inane or patronizing advice, you can restore the balance in your interactions by asking them to tell you of their feelings about your illness. This will clear the air and help put you on an equal footing again.

- Understand that other people may feel threatened by the notion of a debilitating illness that strikes suddenly and without reason. If they deny the reality of your condition, or offer you their ideas for a ready cure, they're doing so out of self-protection. It's too painful to acknowledge that what has happened to you could happen to them or someone else they love. Try to respect how they feel, even as you work toward gaining respect for, and acknowledgment of, *your* feelings.

- None of the psychological mechanisms that may be at play in chronic fatigue syndrome negate the biological reality of the illness. Hold on to this knowledge as you make whatever changes you can in your expectations and lifestyle to promote your own good health.

- If helplessness has become a way of life for you—linked to depression, self-pity, or chronic complaining—then it's time to look for outside support in changing the ways you think about your life.

Dealing With the Realities of CFS

> I felt guilty being a homemaker because I didn't have
> an outside job. So I tried to do even more to make up
> for it: PTA, volunteer teaching, etc.—trying to make
> amends for my being at home. This is the nineties and
> I should be out there. I think society does put a lot of
> pressure on you. You have to be the best and you have
> to be the bravest.

Such messages are very powerful and difficult to resist even
as you make the wrenching readjustment to living with chronic
fatigue syndrome. But you *can* teach yourself to ignore society's
"do-it-all" messages. If you do not ignore them, you may become
much sicker than you thought you could be. I've seen many people
in my practice who are trying to completely deny the illness and
the limitations it imposes. Their suffering is just ruinous as they
alternate between overwork and collapse.

Expectations can grab you at every level, from a simple interaction with a friend to the direction and goals in your life. You've
realized that being a loving spouse, a hardworking employee, or a
selflessly devoted parent and caregiver are all environmental de-
mands that are much more difficult or impossible to maintain. You
may think of your primary role in terms of relationships with others. And those other people have a hard time thinking of you in
any way other than their image of your pre-illness self. You may
not be able to change their thinking, but you can do positive things
for yourself that will release you from impossible expectations.

How Are You?

How do you handle the "How are you's" that people bombard you
with even though you're rarely feeling well?

> People I'm really close to know not to ask. It's become
> like a joke. With people who don't know me, and
> don't know what I face every day, I answer, "Okay."
> Questions about my profession are really painful,
> because that part of my life is quite static right now,

and I don't have much to tell them. So I divert them from those kinds of questions.

When you have chronic fatigue syndrome you learn to identify those people who have the understanding and concern to want to know how you really feel. Some of us hold back our true feelings, because we don't want to be perceived as chronic complainers. It's important, however, to have a confidant or close friend to whom you can express how you really feel. If you don't have such a person in your life, consider going to a local support group meeting or seeing a therapist who is familiar with CFS issues. You may obtain a list of local support groups and counselors from the CFIDS Association of America by calling 1-800-442-3437. If you have the opportunity to share your feelings, your ability to endure the illness improves substantially.

One form of self-disclosure involves asking for help. This is difficult, because many individuals with CFS are used to seeing themselves in the role of giver and helper. They are not used to seeking assistance or being the recipient of care. Try to keep in mind that giving this up is not a show of weakness; rather, it takes courage to seek help, whether in managing household chores, asking for financial assistance, or getting emotional support.

Ask yourself if you would judge someone—say, a disabled person in a wheelchair—who asked others for help. I don't think you would. Yet our high personal standards dictate that we should be able to solve all our problems even when our rational selves tell us that we can't. CFS research scientists cannot yet identify causes or treatments for this illness; is it reasonable to expect yourself to overcome all illness-related difficulties entirely on your own? Your mind can have a powerful influence on how well you cope, but the mind alone cannot banish the limitations brought on by illness. *Realizing your full capacity within the context of your waxing and waning symptoms is a realistic goal.*

Reactions of Family and Friends

The reactions of those close to you can take many forms:

When I first became ill, my husband thought that I would beat this thing. He often said to me, "If I had chronic fatigue syndrome, I'd just ignore the symptoms." But I can't just ignore them. When that fatigue takes over, you've got it. There are other times when he is magnificent and as supportive as he can be. The other person is my mother. She's good, but she doesn't want to face that I'm sick, because I'm her daughter and I'm younger and should be enjoying life. I think it hurts her.

Another woman with CFS tells of a spouse who is desperate for her to get well:

He comes to me all the time saying, "What did the doctor say, what new medicines have you got?" He wants me cured. When I told my husband that I might not be able to return to work, he just went crazy. He thought that in two years I was going to be better. But there is no time prediction with this illness.

People Want To Help You or Cure You

"If you just get rid of your anger, let it go!"

"Couldn't you be a little more positive? You're always complaining."

"Look at the way you eat! Haven't you heard of the yeast-free diet?"

"Get your mind off yourself! If I stayed in bed as much as you did, I'd be sick too."

People close to you, and even total strangers, may offer their own home remedies or personal advice on how to cure you of CFS. Even the most arrogant and patronizing suggestions may be perfectly well-intentioned. Most people don't understand how complex and unyielding the problem really is, nor will they have any idea about how much anguished thought and research you've already done looking for an end to your symptoms.

I can see how difficult it is for people to comprehend our symptoms. One day I was walking up and down the steps like it was nothing, and the next day I was in bed. My mother comes into the room, opens up the drapes. It was a sunny day. She said, "Come on, let's go out for a walk, you'll feel better." And I say, "Walk? You know I can't even get out of bed today." So it upset me because I snapped at her. Did she think I wanted to be in bed on a nice day? I wanted to go Christmas shopping and do so many other things. So she got upset and said, "I don't know how to handle you."

You may find some of the following suggestions useful in dealing with people who try to help you:

- If you know the person well enough, ask about the emotions brought up by your illness. Does the person feel concern, annoyance, discomfort, fear, guilt? Say that you'd really appreciate their honesty in telling you what their reactions are. Tell them that it will help clear the air. You can also say that learning of their feelings will take the pressure off you to pretend to be well, or respond to well-intentioned but worthless advice—"Just eat less chocolate," or "Do volunteer work." Asking other people about their feelings relieves you of the exclusive burden of disclosure: the conversation becomes an exchange instead of a one-way confession.

- When people interact with someone in distress, their impulse is often to try to solve the person's problems immediately instead of really listening and taking in what the distressed person has to say. Most people are uncomfortable with illness—it's too threatening to their own status quo. This may account for the "just world" attitude, which suggests that people "deserve" to be ill as retribution for an unapproved or immoral lifestyle: "Yuppie Flu" is punishment for trying to have it all. No one wants to think that they have no control over the threat of serious illness. It is more comfortable for a healthy person to believe a serious illness such as CFS can be avoided solely through personal choice. The person you speak to may be thinking, "What did he/she do to bring this on? I won't ever allow this to happen to me." The alternative to this kind of magical thinking is to feel vulnerable to the workings of chance, and out of control of one's own health and destiny.

- Your feelings about yourself do not have to be contingent on how someone else reacts to you and your illness. What you think to yourself will determine your emotional reaction to others. You have the choice to recognize that their belief in an instant cure reflects their concern or discomfort, but has nothing to do with you; or you can focus on how helpless and misunderstood you feel.

- Many—perhaps most—people with CFS have read books on mind/body cures. We've tried numerous medical and alternative therapies. We've worked very hard to become the "exceptional patients" who allegedly cure themselves through pure determination and will. Even though we may have learned techniques and strategies that help us, there is no evidence that we can cure ourselves—no evidence at all. It's unfair to expect others to understand this unless you explain it to them; and many people will be unwilling to accept what you say. They need to distance themselves from your illness, because its present status as "incurable" is just too threatening. Creating distance is how they cope.

CFS: Escape From Responsibility?

Drs. Susan Abbey and Paul Garfinkel (1991) suggested in a controversial article published in *The American Journal of Psychiatry* that chronic fatigue syndrome is a socially sanctioned form of illness behavior that allows the sufferer to be excused from the responsibilities of work, family, and social involvement. The "primary gain" is relief from responsibility, to use the psychological jargon. The supposed secondary gain is the attention, care, and support received for being ill. Thus a very neatly packaged psychosocial explanation for CFS was legitimized in the scientific literature. Dr. Abbey further suggested that the American cultural expectation for women to achieve in all life domains creates an overwhelming pressure from which they escape into chronic fatigue syndrome.

Of course, all illness and disease is expressed in a social and cultural context, which gives meaning to the specific illness. Chronic fatigue syndrome is no exception. Dr. Abbey's argument appears to rest on the assumption that no biological factor will be found in CFS, and therefore we must explain CFS symptoms as a purely cultural phenomenon unworthy of serious scientific scrutiny. It is hard to fathom how any physician or health practitioner who has had extensive experience with patients suffering from CFS could dismiss the reality of the illness with such a facile, unsupported explanation.

We can define important psychological issues in CFS without negating biological mechanisms. Positive lifestyle changes *can* result from the CFS experience. People do reevaluate their life priorities and commitments when they're restricted by any chronic illness: their knowledge of their limitations allows them to pursue what is most important and to avoid wasting time on trivialities. In this sense, a primary "gain" from the illness is the reassertion of control—the choice to live a more manageable and healthier life that deliberately emphasizes personal well-being as a goal.

But redirecting our lives does not invalidate our illness, our feelings, or the painful reality of our symptoms. In my treatment of patients with other fatiguing illnesses, such as multiple sclerosis and lupus, I've noticed that similar processes of readjustment and redirection take place. But at no point are these patients intellectually and emotionally abandoned by their physicians in the way in which people with CFS have been. It seems that until a biological identifier is found, chronic fatigue syndrome will be an "orphan illness" that must go begging for research funds, professional recognition, and public acceptance. This reality highlights the importance of networking, self-support, and political advocacy among the people who suffer from the illness and the people who care for them.

Redefining our priorities is a frustrating exercise. Many people with chronic fatigue syndrome—although not necessarily a majority—find it difficult if not impossible to modify their high standards of personal performance: they feel impelled to do for others, they have difficulty saying no, give too much, and consequently have little left over for themselves. These personality traits may or may not describe you. It's possible that you feel a certain "relief" from responsibility due to the disabling effects of CFS. I think it's important to at least ask yourself these difficult questions about the meaning of CFS in your life.

This is not to imply in any sense that your CFS burden is not legitimate or real. What it does say is that powerful social norms can encourage "health-hazardous" behavior and lifestyles (Ware 1993). A harried and frenetic lifestyle may be one factor in the mix of biological, social, and psychological factors that combine to produce chronic fatigue syndrome.

Illness Behavior in CFS

Rarely do I see the individual with CFS who adopts "responsibility avoidance" as a major role. Our achievement motivation would not allow it. However, we do have a chronic disabling condition, so it is legitimate to ask ourselves if we have adopted the role of invalid as an "alternative lifestyle."

Due to our limitations, we are not the autonomous people we used to be. We are often forced to ask for and receive help for things that we could previously do for ourselves. It's important to tell yourself that this dependence on other individuals is not a disgrace. Every individual with chronic fatigue syndrome will acknowledge assuming the "helpless" role at times. It is not a crime to acknowledge such illness behavior. I fall into it sometimes; you may as well. However, if helplessness has become a way of life for you—linked to depression, self-pity, or chronic complaining—then it's time to look for outside help in changing the ways you think about your life.

Finally, I believe it's absurd to suggest that CFS symptoms are a socially acceptable way to avoid responsibility. The enduring skepticism of family, friends, and physicians would hardly suggest a social "sanction." Do some people with CFS "enjoy" primary and secondary gains of being ill? Perhaps one in twenty whom I have seen appear to accept the illness a little too readily, and show a surprising resignation to their symptoms. (Of course, it's also possible that they *are* ill and accepting it.) The great majority, however, are desperate to get well. They spend thousands of dollars on traditional and alternative medical treatments, change their diets, travel vast distances to seek out any promising new treatment, and generally "doctor-shop" for years. The results of their efforts are often frustration and disappointment. Do these people want to be ill? I don't think so.

Step 3

Create Well-Being: The Relaxation Benefit

Coping Strategies in a Nutshell

- Twenty minutes a day of relaxation practice can make you feel better. There are several proven methods for inducing a state of relaxation and peace. Whatever method you use, the end result will be an enhanced ability to cope with the symptoms of chronic fatigue syndrome, more restful periods of sleep, less confusion, and more clarity in your thinking.

- Use the word *relax* as a way to induce relaxation—inhale as you say the first syllable in your mind, then exhale with the second syllable.

- Creative visualization is another way to rid yourself of stress, and induce a relaxed state of body and mind.

- Progressive muscle relaxation offers the advantage of a re- flexive, automatic release of tension.

- Healing imagery is another technique that has been shown to promote stress relief and well-being.

How Relaxation Can Help You

As little as 20 minutes a day of relaxation practice can have powerful health-inducing effects. Relaxation practice will:

- Dissipate the accumulated tensions of the day

- Reduce your anxiety and worry

- Create a sense of well-being

- Help you cope with stress

- Give you a sense of control over symptoms as well as your reactions to them

- Improve the restfulness of your sleep

There are other important physical benefits of daily relaxation. Several recent studies have shown improvements in immune functioning among healthy individuals who practice relaxation twice daily. After 15 years of doing meditative relaxation, I know firsthand the psychological and physical benefits of the technique. The main benefit for me is a nearly constant feeling of ease, comfort, and serenity that years of meditation have produced. The relaxed feeling also buffers the negative effects of stress and day-to-day upsets. You can begin to achieve these results with only a few days to a few weeks of daily practice.

The advantage of self-relaxation is its simplicity. People sometimes dismiss it—"How can something this simple produce a positive result? What I need is a powerful drug." But we've all tried drugs, and have rarely found them to be helpful. They may temporarily reduce some of the symptoms of CFS, but often have disturbing side effects. As you are well aware, many people with CFS are drug-sensitive and cannot tolerate standard doses of medication. Relaxation offers long-term, chemical-free benefits.

Obstacles to Relaxation

If you have many responsibilities, it may be very difficult to put aside time to relax or meditate. Even in your fatigued, less capable condition, relaxation may seem to be something you shouldn't indulge in because it's a "waste" of time. Your energy may be at such a premium that when you do have the get-up-and-go to do something, you don't want to waste it on something as "unproductive" as sitting still—after all, you have a full schedule of things you'd like to get done! Merely thinking about doing something may feel more "constructive" than practicing relaxation.

Even after many years of practice, it can still be difficult for me to find the patience for focused relaxation. Especially if you have a family, there may be almost constant distractions in your household. One person with CFS told me of her own unique approach to relaxing with the family around:

> I've learned to relax even when there are distractions.
> In fact, I've tried it at the dinner table when my
> husband and the kids are fighting with each other. I
> just close my eyes. I feel tense in my chest a lot. If I
> just concentrate on letting go, the relaxation begins to
> take hold no matter how much commotion there is. I
> concentrate on the "re-lax" phrase as you taught us.
> Just concentrating on that word starts to produce the
> feeling. My kids began to get the signal that as soon as
> I close my eyes, they aren't going to get any attention
> from me for fighting. Actually, they're probably so
> used to getting a rise from me that when I do
> something quite different they say to themselves,
> "What's going on?" I think it diverts them from their
> fighting or whatever else it is that has them so wound
> up. So even in the midst of high stress you can take
> time and do that re-lax phrase.

A set of positive affirmations can facilitate your relaxation. Affirmations are succinct, positive statements that you repeat to yourself at different times throughout the day as a way of adjusting your mind to their truth and feasibility. It's not necessary that you really believe them at the outset. Try these self-statements as a way to help yourself overcome personal obstacles to relaxation:

- I'm entitled to take time for myself.

- Relaxation will improve my mood and my coping ability.

- Relaxation benefits myself and those around me—that makes sense.

- Relaxation will make me more efficient.

Relaxation Techniques

I teach a very simple, straightforward relaxation method to my groups. Sit in a comfortable chair—often a recliner is best. Say to yourself silently, "Re-," as you inhale, and "lax" as you exhale. Choose a comfortable, quiet setting, and minimize distractions as much as possible. Let the answering machine take phone calls or turn off the ringer. If you have young children, wait until they're napping or put them in another room with their favorite video and a supply of juice and snacks. Settle yourself far enough away not to be bothered by the noise, but close enough to stay attuned to an emergency. Practice the *re-lax* phrase for two 10-minute periods a day, once in the morning and once in the afternoon, preferably before meals—but make sure you're not uncomfortably hungry. In just the first few days, you may start to feel a difference. You'll be able to release tension and stress; over the long haul, you may discover that a sense of well-being is possible even though you're ill.

Visualization

Visualization involves the use of your imagination to achieve a state of relaxation. The first step is to select a calming scene to focus on—perhaps a vacation spot where you've relaxed easily in the past, or even a place you remember fondly from childhood. Anything goes here: you can construct a place completely from scratch if you want to, or create a composite of the most wonderful and serene places you've ever visited. In my experience, the most popular locations for a calming visualization are the beach, the country, and the mountains, in that order.

To make your imaginative journey as vivid as possible, write down a description of your calming scene. Make sure you fill in as much detail as possible, using all five senses. What are the sights, sounds, smells, tastes, and textures there? After you've written your notes, sit in a comfortable chair and create the scene in your mind over a 10- to 15-minute period. Let yourself become completely absorbed in the details; let yourself be transported by them until you begin to relax emotionally and physically.

Here's a sample beach scene you could use. If you prefer, ask a friend who has a soothing voice to dictate this description onto audiotape, and then play it back while relaxing with closed eyes.

> Imagine yourself spending an afternoon at the beach.
> The sand feels warm and soft against your skin.
> You are sitting on the sand observing the ocean, the
> azure blue water; viewing the flow of the waves as
> they move rhythmically to the shore, the water
> becoming a light transparent green as it flows to the
> shoreline. And you see the whitecaps on the waves as
> the waves roll onto the shore; yes, waves gently
> reaching the shore, like sparkling water spilling on the
> sand, feeling a salty, refreshing spray in the air, that
> refreshing misty spray permeating your body—so
> wonderfully invigorating and uplifting; revitalizing
> and relaxing.

> Allow yourself the next few moments to imagine the
> pleasant flow of the waves onto the shore as they rise
> and fall, rise and fall. Go ahead now and imagine the
> waves. (Pause for about 15 seconds.)

> Alright. Very good. Now you decide to take an easy
> stroll along the beach as you view the surf; yes,
> observe the curving shoreline off in the distance, the
> curving shoreline as it merges with the horizon.
> As you walk onward, onward, you feel the sand
> crunching beneath your feet; such a pleasant
> sensation—the warm crunchy sand. It complements
> the warmth of the sun overhead. Feel the warmth of
> the sun on your back, that gentle warmth flowing
> down your back and throughout your body;
> comfortable warmth from the sun filling you with
> pleasant sensations. With your senses so very

aware, you notice the sand dunes rising along the beach, sand dunes with isolated clumps of tall grass on their slopes. Noticing the tall grass gently swaying in the breeze. The breezes creating tranquil feelings.

And as you walk onward, you hear the sound of seagulls in the distance. A flock of white seagulls approaching, flying so easily, gliding in the wind, making their distinctive squeaking sounds passing overhead. Now flying off in the distance, leaving you with a feeling of serenity. . . . You feel a gentle breeze at your back. The gentle breeze coaxing you further along, heightening your senses.

Now, as you look across the waves, you see a sleek white sailboat moving through the water. The boat moving so gracefully, the sails filled with gently sweeping winds. Enjoy the silent steadiness of the boat as it moves along with the wind.

Now as you gaze further toward the horizon, you see the sun setting. Yes, the sun setting in a full display of vivid colors: bright yellows, deep reds, and burnt oranges against the light gray clouds and a pale blue sky. The sun descends, projecting a long wedge of yellow light across the water; slowly sinking down . . . A breathtaking serenity begins to pervade the atmosphere. An emerging serenity so deep that it is fully absorbing your senses.

Now you begin to conclude the experience—finish the experience with acceptance and peace, acceptance and peace . . . Allow yourself the next minute, all the time in the world, all the time you need to bring yourself back to wakefulness, your eyes opening slowly, feeling relaxed and refreshed.

You may find this beach image helpful in your daily relaxation sessions.

Progressive Muscle Relaxation

If you've tried the *re-lax* phrase and the visualization image without significant relaxation, I would suggest progressive muscle relaxation as your next alternative. The advantage of this exercise is that it produces a reflexive, automatic release of tension. Also, there is a minimum amount of mental focusing or attention required.

Progressive muscle relaxation involves tensing and then relaxing different muscle groups. As you tense and then relax each muscle group, experience the localized release of tension. Feel the contrast between the tension and the release of tension. Some muscle groups will release in a much more obvious manner than others—these may represent your personal stress points. For instance, you may find that the jaw muscle releases to a much greater degree than the other muscle groups. Your jaw may be the place in your body where you harbor tension anger, frustration, fear, or stress in general.

If you experience only mild relaxed feelings after completing the sequence, and feel up to it, repeat the entire exercise to deepen the relaxation.

If any one of these exercises causes or increases pain, simply skip it and go on to the next one. Keep each muscle group tensed for about the number of seconds specified in parentheses—it's not important to be precise here. People usually do these exercises in a sitting position but a lying-down position is just as effective.

Follow these instructions for progressive relaxation:

Arms: Raise your arms from your sides, make fists, and tense up all the muscles from your fingers to your biceps (8 sec). Release the tension in your arms, let them drop down, and experience the sense of relaxation in all the muscles that were tensed before (15 sec).

Shoulders: Raise your shoulders into a high shrug. Feel tension across the shoulders and back of the neck (8 sec). Release and feel the relaxed sensations (15 sec).

Jaw: Press your molars together—not too hard—to clench the muscles of your jaw. Feel the tension (8 sec). Then release (15 sec).

Eyes: Open your eyes very wide, raise your eyebrows, and wrinkle up your forehead (8 sec). Release the eye muscles to a resting comfortable position. Keep your focus soft, if your eyes are open, and your forehead smooth (15 sec). Close your eyes very tightly (8 sec). Then release the tension, eyes returning to a comfortable position (15 sec).

Legs: (If sitting) Push the soles of your feet directly into the floor. Feel the tension in your leg muscles, from your feet up through your calves and thighs (8 sec). Then release (15 sec). (If lying down) Tense your legs (your feet will rise slightly) (8 sec). Then release (15 sec).

You can use these exercises in conjunction with the *re-lax* phrase. After completing the full sequence of muscle relaxation exercises, think to yourself *"re-"* when you inhale and *"lax"* as you exhale (5 min). You'll come to associate the relaxed feelings created through progressive muscle relaxation with the *re-lax* phrase itself. With repetition, you'll find that just thinking the *re-lax* phrase will produce feelings of relaxation.

As you practice progressive relaxation you'll become more aware of how personal stress in your daily life affects your muscles. Perhaps you'll feel your shoulders rising and your neck stiffening, or your forehead tensing, in moments of stress. As you become more aware of these physical responses to stress, you can learn to release these tense muscles just as you do during the progressive relaxation exercise: and you'll feel calmer as a result. If one of your chronic fatigue symptoms is muscle aches, you may experience some relief as the progressive relaxation lessens your muscular tension. If you experience muscle pain, the voluntary skeletal muscles may reflexively tense in response to that pain. Progressive relaxation can alleviate habitual muscle tension and give you a sense of control over it.

Relaxation Tape

If the above methods do not work for you, or if you would like to enhance your relaxation experience, you can order an audio cassette tape that I've specially prepared for people who have chronic fatigue syndrome. (Ordering information may be found at

the end of this book.) The tape contains deep relaxation suggestions with interspersed coping messages. The recorded relaxation
instructions may be more powerful, because they allow you to focus outside yourself—away from the stress and symptoms you normally feel. Based on the feedback I've received, the tape is very
likely to work for you, even if your personal attempts to use relaxation techniques haven't.

Relaxation as a Coping Skill

The daily stress you experience in relation to family, work,
and social involvements may be reduced by the focused applica-
tion of relaxation methods. Use relaxation techniques as a coping
skill when stress levels begin to rise. Become aware of the early
signs of stressful feelings, such as a mild headache, stiffness in the
neck, a nervous or tight feeling in your stomach, a jittery sensation,
a restless feeling, or whatever your physical reaction might be. Begin to identify these premonitory signals, and use your relaxation
techniques when you first notice feelings of stress coming on. Controlling these initial symptoms will be far more effective than coping with stress that has become intense and overwhelming.

Understand that persistent stress may create its own fatigue
and merge with your CFS experience. I'm not even remotely suggesting that stress is the central issue in CFS; but it may be the one
class of symptoms that you can minimize through behavioral techniques.

Relaxation and Sleep Hygiene

The immune system is repaired or bolstered during sleep, and
it also has a role in regulating sleep. Short-term sleep deprivation
in healthy individuals can cause the immune system to go into
overdrive (as if fighting off an illness), and also cause daytime fatigue. This finding suggests that our disturbed sleep patterns may
result in a state of chronic sleep deprivation, which influences immune function and contributes to the severity of our symptoms.

If your sleep is disturbed in any way—if you have trouble
falling asleep or staying asleep, wake too early, have bad dreams
or unrestful sleep—relaxation can promote more restorative and

restful patterns. At bedtime, practice the *re-lax* phrase while you're in bed. If you have trouble falling asleep, the *re-lax* phrase can replace your usual worries, regrets, or planning thoughts about the coming day. Using the phrase will distract you from those sleep-defeating thoughts and engender a sleep-inducing calm. Repeat the *re-lax* phrase in your mind, following your breathing, until you fall asleep.

If staying asleep is the problem, relaxation practice at bedtime will program your mind and body to get more restful sleep. Pre-sleep relaxation thoughts have a powerful influence on the depth and duration of your sleep. If you wake up during the night, use the *re-lax* phrase to purge your frustration or anxiety, or dispel unsettled feelings about bad dreams. If you don't return to sleep right away, you'll at least feel calmer, which is much more restorative than lying in bed with feelings of stress or tension.

In addition to internal stress, become aware of sleep inhibitors in your environment. You may be a more sensitive sleeper with your illness than you used to be. Are low-level noises interfering with your sleep? Your spouse may be turning over in bed or snoring. The sound of the television from another room, or even the background noise level, may interfere with your sleep patterns. Recognize that noise lessens the depth of sleep. Possible remedies include the use of ear plugs, or sleeping in a separate bed in a quiet room. I find the soft, foam-type earplugs to be quite helpful. Sometimes a white noise machine, which makes a shooshing sound, can also mask disturbing sounds in your home. If you're hypersensitive to light, make sure that your bedroom is fully darkened before going to sleep. If your mattress isn't comfortable—if it's too hard, too soft, or uneven—get a new one that suits you better. You can firm up an overly soft mattress by putting a board underneath, or soften up a hard mattress with one of the egg-crate foam pads developed for hospital use, but now available in any bedding store or large department store (these pads usually cost less than $30).

The principles of sleep hygiene involve altering your bedtime habits so that they're more conducive to sleep. Use your bed only for sleep at night and not for other activities such as television watching, reading, or work. This will help you associate restful sleep with your bed. Long periods of daytime rest and sleep in your bed can actually make you more susceptible to depression, and can interfere with your sleep at night.

Allow yourself a wind-down period before going to bed. During the pre-sleep hour, engage in activities that you know are going to make you sleepy, and refrain from mental and physical activity that stimulates you. Don't exercise or eat a large meal just before bed. If energy permits, sex can help relax you, release tension, and actually promote sleep, as long as you feel perfectly safe and comfortable with your partner. A hot bath before bed or a light snack containing calcium may also be sleep-inducing.

Another important factor in promoting restful sleep is establishing and maintaining a daily routine of low-level mental and physical activities that help you differentiate daytime activity from sleep at night. Don't wear pajamas or your bathrobe during the day. Develop a ritual for getting ready for bed at night.

> As a result of efforts to improve my sleep, I have gone
> from being nearly bedfast and severely dependent on
> others in 1988, to functioning at a semi-dependent
> level. This means I can now do some of the simpler
> activities of daily living, but still depend on others for
> ones requiring more strength, stamina, and endurance.
> The progress I have made has been slow and gradual,
> *not* quick or dramatic. However, it has made it
> possible for me to maintain some degree of steadiness
> and predictability in my energy levels, to regain some
> independence and self-sufficiency, and to do some
> of the activities which formally were impossible.
> (Keim 1994)

Relaxing Away Your Headache

CFS is characterized by a pressure-like headache that appears to be intrinsic to the illness. Daily relaxation as described above will produce some alleviation of that pressure headache. If you experience migraine headaches, relaxation can be helpful *if it is used at the earliest sign of an oncoming headache.* Learn to recognize those early signals, such as a knot in the back of your neck, a tense feeling in your jaw, or, in the case of some types of migraine headache, tearing eyes, nausea, or such visual irregularities as a perception of flashing lights. A large dose of relaxation at this time may well reduce the severity of the headache.

For mild to moderate tension headaches, relaxation may alleviate the entire headache. In order to get maximum headache relief, daily practice of relaxation is recommended. Then, if the headache occurs, you'll be prepared to achieve a relaxation response and counteract the pain. With extended use of daily relaxation you may find that the frequency, severity, and duration of your headaches decline as well. These improvements are due to the effects of generalized calm, which minimizes the stress and tension that can trigger a headache.

Relaxation as a Worry Reducer

Worry thoughts are often prefaced with "What if," or "Suppose . . ." or "Oh my God. . . ." Worry is sustained by a devout belief in the possibility of disaster and defeat. If you were a worrier before your illness, you're probably worrying even more now that you have the added burden of CFS. Or perhaps your patterns of worrying started with the onset of CFS, as a result of all the new difficulties you faced.

Whatever the source of your worry—whether it be money, work, family issues, friends, or an uncertain future—you can learn to worry less. Relaxation is a straightforward method to interrupt and reduce worried thoughts. Say the *re-lax* phrase when you find yourself caught in a worry pattern.

> Last night I started to feel my symptoms come on quickly, with nausea, dry mouth, and fatigue. I lay down and said to myself: "Okay. My panic starts to come when I feel fatigued, but I'll just lie here and say 're-lax.'" And when I did, the symptoms lessened.

> I had to go into traffic and pick up my husband, run home, take a bath, and come here. I was at the light getting stressed out with all the things I had to do and worrying about whether I could do it all, how I would

feel and everything. So at the light, I just kept saying to myself "re-lax," and it helped reduce the anxiety about everything I had to do, the fear I wouldn't be able to do it, and whether I would be fatigued, and it really did help.

There is more about worry control in Step 5.

Less Confusion, More Clarity With Relaxation

Cognitive problems are perhaps the most frustrating and de-bilitating symptoms of chronic fatigue syndrome. At a recent CFS conference, several individuals told me that their daily relaxation alleviated their cognitive confusion and distractability. It's certainly worthwhile to experiment with relaxation: see if you can diminish the cognitive confusion. If your confusion lessens, you'll be able to focus your thoughts with more clarity and precision.

Overall, relaxation has powerful stress-reducing properties. With regular practice of relaxation techniques, increased awareness of stress triggers, and use of relaxation skills whenever stress or symptoms arise, your sense of self-control and well-being will sig-nificantly improve.

Healing Imagery

The technique of healing imagery has often been cited in the psy-chological literature on treatment of cancer (Siegel 1986). The ill-ness outcome data suggest that coping relaxation, as described above, and healing imagery are both effective in promoting well-being, stress relief, and symptom control. You can use the above relaxation methods or healing imagery, whichever you prefer, and achieve similar results. Some people with chronic fatigue syndrome find healing imagery to be a good way to "fight back" during set-backs or relapses.

Healing imagery involves visualizing the immune system or other physiological mechanisms which, if harnessed and strength-ened via imagery, lead to symptom relief in chronic illness. The following healing imagery script involves a sequence of relaxation suggestions, coping metaphors for the CFS experience, calming ideas to release stress, and healing imagery that promotes physical and emotional strengthening.

You might want to record the script on tape and then play it back to yourself. Sit in a comfortable chair or recliner, or lie down—whatever feels right to you.

If you don't want to listen to your own voice, I would suggest asking someone who you do not know very well to dictate the imagery onto a cassette tape. This individual would preferably have a pleasant voice and speak slowly to maximize the effect. Or you can order my prerecorded tape. Ordering information is available at the end of this book. Asking a family member or friend whom you know very well to tape the exercise may not work as well, because your feelings toward that person may interfere with the relaxation process. When you have the tape ready, play it once a day to reinforce its healing messages.

Relaxation Suggestions

One, let your eyes close. Two, take a long, deep breath, and three, slowly release the breath. Feel the release, the letting go as you exhale and allow your breathing to assume an easy, natural rhythm. Focus on the easy breathing rhythm . . . inhale and exhale. You need not control your breathing in any way; simply observe it and recognize it as a natural process, an easy response and a source of relaxation . . . Observation is not concentration, but simply passive attention to your own natural rhythms. Appreciate them . . . Now focus on the release of breath. Each time you exhale, you release tension as well as breathe. With each exhale, there is a perceptible release of tension, as well as breath. Exhale, release; exhale, release . . . Feel the release, the letting go that accompanies each release of breath. Exhale, release . . . Now allowing relaxed feelings to radiate upward . . . to the shoulders, going across the shoulders and descending through both arms. Upper arms relaxed . . . lower arms relaxed . . . both arms relaxing. Now relaxed feelings descending through the chest, flowing into the stomach, the stomach becoming relaxed. Relaxed sensations spreading through the hips and to the upper legs and enveloping the upper legs. Now flowing to the lower legs . . . all the way down to the feet. The feet becoming loose and relaxed, loose and relaxed. Relaxed sensations retracing their gentle path upward. Lower legs relaxed . . . upper legs relaxed. Relaxed feelings ascending the lower back, lower back loosening . . . Now proceeding to the upper back . . . up the back of the neck . . . infusing the area with relaxed sensations. Now spreading up over the scalp and down the face . . . forehead relaxed, eyes relaxed, jaw becoming loose, limp, and slack; loose, limp, and slack.

You have reached a pleasant plateau of calm and comfort—recognize the feelings you now have. Know that you can reproduce these feelings with regular, easy practice . . .

Now, as I count from one to ten, you can feel even more relaxed: 1, more relaxed; 2, even more; 3, deeper down; 4, more relaxed; 5, calmer still; 6, even more; 7, deeper down; 8, more relaxed; 9, so very calm; 10, your entire physical self completely immersed in relaxed sensations . . . calm, wavy, deep relaxation, so deeply and comfortably relaxed.

Coping Metaphors

Now, ease the pounding of your heart by the quieting of your mind. Steady your pace with the vision of the eternal reach of time—yes . . . feeling within the confusion of your day the calmness of *the* everlasting hills. Release the tensions of your nerves and muscles with the soothing music of the singing streams that live in your memory. Allow yourself the art of mini vacations, of slowing down to look at a flower, to chat with a friend, to pat a dog, to read a few lines from a good book, to fish, to dream. Remind yourself each day of the fable of the hare and the tortoise, so that you may know that the race is not always to the swift, that there is more in life than increasing speed. Look upward into the branches of the towering oak and know that it grew great and strong because it grew slowly and well. It inspires you to send your roots deep into the soil of life's enduring values, so that you may grow upward toward the stars of your greater destiny (Tubesing and Tubesing 1983, p. 80-81).

Letting Go of Stress

Now, let your thoughts continue. Yes, you need not interrupt the flow of your thoughts. That natural flow of inner experience can be used to engender calm and peace. Your thoughts may be pleasant or unpleasant, relaxing or tensing. And it makes no difference, no difference because your thoughts will harmonize with your inner experience. Yes, harmonize so closely that thoughts will become free of stress. Free of tension . . . by harmonizing with your inner experience. By flowing with it. Your experience is a medium through which thoughts will flow easily . . . naturally. Your experience transported effortlessly, guided through a smooth, harmonious background of floating sensations; releasing restrictions and opening awareness. Yes, floating, as your thoughts loosen . . . loosen from any rigid pattern. Feel the freeing of those patterns as the easy flow guides your experience to a new openness . . . obstacles fall away as you recognize that no goal need be achieved. There is no calculation or concentration, only the increasing realization of calm . . . yes, your thoughts are becoming part of that gentle background . . . flowing so naturally with it, floating easily . . . that comfortable drift is all you need to relax and release, relax and release.

Feel the floating sensation as you imagine yourself floating, drifting. Your entire body floating—thoughts, feelings, sensations, so comfortably afloat, all the time recognizing your power to create this relaxed state of being. Your power to draw upon those internal images. The vast reservoir of imagination available to create and sustain floating calm. Now let us raise your floating awareness even more, enhance your floating experience. Imagine yourself floating on a cloud; yes . . . use this image to create further calm. An image of a cloud, a fluffy, white, powder-puff of a cloud. Embellish the cloud however you wish . . . and gently sustain the image in your own mind, that's right, sustain the image in your own mind right now.

Healing Imagery

Your healing can now begin, yes, your healing begins from within yourself. An inner radiance that begins as a mere speck of light, yes, an inner point of light and warmth . . . radiating strength and power . . . yes, the strength and power that grows warm and radiant . . . inner strength. Feel it, experience it fully, thoroughly, inner radiance growing stronger . . . Ready now, yes ready to direct its healing strength towards your weakened system. Yes, the inner radiance directing its strength towards your body. Feel that inner sense of strength beginning, working within your body. Feeling revitalized, re-energized . . . strengthening as your inner radiance strengthens and energizes. Feel the warm, intense energy doing its work; reactivating, restoring your body . . . yes, restoring your body. Experience that strengthening fully, thoroughly, that inner boosting, growing even stronger now, stronger, more powerful than before. And as you feel that strength, you believe in yourself and your ability to succeed in your goal of rebuilding your body. Yes, believing in the strength of your thoughts, images, and the totality of your internal powers. You believe so strongly, feeling that boost even now, yes, yet remaining tolerant, letting time pass, knowing that any worthwhile goal takes time, any worthwhile goal. And you have resolved to accomplish your goal, believing you can . . . re-energizing, boosting your system. You hold firmly to that belief; yes, so firmly . . . feeling less fatigued . . . and this message remains with you, far beyond these words, far beyond these words. Now, slowly bringing yourself back to wakefulness, eyes opening gradually, feeling relaxed and refreshed.

Step 4

Pace Yourself

Coping Strategies in a Nutshell

- You can function with your limited energy if you modify your behavioral goals: keep your plans modest and flexible.

- Get the rest you need, but allow yourself time and opportunity to do things you enjoy.

- Try an experiment of reducing your activity level, then very gradually building it again. Some studies claim that a gradual buildup of activity and exercise can alleviate depression and modulate some symptoms of CFS. Alternatively, you may find that you've just been trying to do too much, and that you can function better in general with a lower level of activity. There is no one answer that's right for everyone.

We're not used to pacing ourselves. Our habit was to fill up our daily schedule, then add a few more activities, do two things at once whenever possible, and hurry, if not run, from one activity to the next. You may even have enjoyed the frenetic pace—I did. But now we're paying dearly for doing too much. If you felt like a Formula I racing car before, you may feel as if you're now performing more like a VW Beetle in low gear.

But you can function with your limited energy if you modify your behavioral goals. Of course, your energy reserves may fluctuate enormously from day to day, or week to week. Because there is so little "up time" and so much "down time," you probably want to maximize activity when you do have energy. I'm reluctant to tell people to pace themselves when they're feeling better, because they usually ignore me. When your energy level is between the extremes of vigor and collapse, it's difficult to predict how much you can do. You don't want to do something if you think it's going to make you collapse. On the other hand, if you avoid the activity, you don't know if you would have collapsed. An activity that is well tolerated on one occasion may lead to a debilitating symptom flare-up at other times. With CFS, our bias always leads us to try to do more. So, generally, I don't say, "Look, you probably could do more than you are doing"; because people with CFS are usually doing more than they should be doing already (while attempting to ignore their symptoms).

Pacing Suggestions

First of all, keep your plans modest and flexible. A 43-year-old woman with CFS uses this strategy:

> I never plan very far in the future anymore. I just go
> week by week. I do have long-term goals, but I'm not
> in a big hurry to get to them. I didn't ask for this
> illness, and I don't know what God is going to hand
> me in the future. Maybe I'll get real sick again; maybe
> I'll run six miles three times a week like I used to. I
> don't know; but I won't multiply expectations in
> myself to do that. It only adds pressure.

In addition to flexible planning and goals, CFS patients need rest—perhaps "aggressive rest," as some have termed the phrase. Rest allows time for modest physical restoration. After you do self-relaxation, allow yourself to lie down for a brief interval; or take a nap. As you schedule rest intervals, you're acknowledging to yourself that symptoms usually can be ignored only up to a certain point before they catch up with you. The following individual with CFS gives herself the time she needs to rest and restore her energy:

> When I'm so fatigued and can't do much, what I can do is make the best of how I'm feeling and try to nurture myself—like I was a little kid who is sick. So maybe I'll drive to this little town two minutes away and get a new video. I'll turn the lights off and I'll light candles. I get my favorite comforter out, put my Teddy bear next to me on the couch, and treat myself. Now I want this to be perfectly understood. This isn't wanting to be ill; but rather than plaguing myself with all the things I can't do, and beating myself up, I nurture myself instead. When I'm feeling ill and exhausted, I create that same situation and positive feeling. It isn't a sad feeling.

Pacing yourself also means allowing yourself time to do things you enjoy. Of course even enjoyable events expend your limited energies. You might well ask yourself: "Am I willing to pay the price in symptoms to do something I'd really enjoy?" This is always a personal choice. I don't believe that any doctor, therapist, or anyone else knows better than you do how much activity you can handle. The following thoughts from a 26-year-old woman illustrate how arduous the decision to do something can be:

> I was afraid to be asked out to do anything, because if I had to say "No," they'd think of me in a negative way. I sang in the church choir, and I used to do musical theater. I haven't done any of that since I became ill. It's only in the last six months that I've been feeling consistently better than I was at the beginning. Now when I do commit it's really intense

for me. I feel this sense of accomplishment. It's like a little milestone.

With fewer activities on your schedule, you can be more selective about choosing what might have the most personal benefit for you.

Even after I do enjoyable things, I'm still tired; but sometimes it's worth having some really tired, tired days after you do stuff you enjoy.

You learn to negotiate and compromise with yourself:

I've learned to moderate my enjoyments. Now I don't go out and work hard for five or six hours at a stretch. I work for two or three hours, and to me that's better, because I don't have to take a week off to recover.

Here's how I've adapted to my exercise limitations.

I've had to learn to pace myself with aerobic exercise, something I used to enjoy immensely—perhaps to the point of fanatical obsession. I thought of my several-times-a-week jogging activity as the key to my immortality. My aerobics would keep me alive until I was 1,000 years old. Clearly I had to compromise on that fantasy. Now I'm walking three times a week, two miles each time, if I can handle it. With the latest research on physical activity suggesting that just walking about doing your daily tasks can sustain healthy fitness, I feel encouraged.

Exercise and CFS: The Research

The role of exercise in CFS rehabilitation has become a controversial issue. A cognitive-behavioral treatment study of 27 CFS patients conducted by Dr. S. Butler and his colleagues (1991) reported that one-third of the subjects became symptom-free after a course of behavioral intervention. The therapy involved scheduling a series of increasingly vigorous activities to overcome an alleged fear of symptom activation. These authors believe that CFS begins as an infectious illness, but is psychologically maintained by the fear of fatigue symptom flare-ups. It follows from this logic that teaching the patients to become more active and overcome their fears can make them well, or can at least greatly improve their condition.

There are problems and shortcomings in this study. First, there was a high dropout rate (31%), which may have created an atypical sample of people with chronic fatigue syndrome. Secondly, there was no control group that would have helped to understand the reported results. Finally, the treatment was given over a period of several months, so it's possible that some of the patients would have had remissions with or without treatment.

A second study (Lloyd et al. 1993) failed to replicate the above findings: a similar treatment involving a gradual increase in physical activity was no more effective than a placebo or transfer factor (an immunomodulatory drug) in ameliorating stress, depression, or CFS symptoms, or in increasing physical activity. None of the three treatment conditions produced significant improvements in the CFS patients.

I conducted a third cognitive-behavioral study (Friedberg and Krupp 1994) that used stress management and coping techniques for people with chronic fatigue syndrome participating in therapy groups. To allow us to compare therapy techniques with the other two studies, a graduated activity intervention was also scheduled. When I presented the idea of setting up 10 behavioral targets, or goals, that each person wanted to achieve, I received immediate and forceful objections to this approach. Almost unanimously, my patients stated that they were already exhausting themselves by doing as much as they could. How could they possibly set up behavioral goals requiring even more exertion? These people were highly motivated, responsible individuals—not a self-pitying group that would reject helpful suggestions. Their test scores did not indicate that they were afraid of doing more. Importantly, a full 75 percent of them strongly agreed with the statement, "I would like to do more, but my fatigue limits me." Overall I found no sound reason to doubt their motivation to respond to useful suggestions. Given these considerations, I withdrew graduated activity as a treatment intervention.

Instead of generally avoiding activity, these individuals had to selectively choose activities that did not deplete their limited energies. Rather than fearing symptom flare-ups, the people in my study were *frustrated* by their symptoms. Stress management and coping techniques produced a trend towards reduced levels of depression, and significant declines in negative thinking about fatigue symptoms. The greatest improvements occurred in the most depressed individuals, who showed significant changes on measures of depression, stress, and even fatigue. However, their fatigue levels remained abnormally high, despite the improvement. In my judgment, these findings reflect the benefits of cognitive-behavioral stress management, not as a cure, but rather as a way to ameliorate and cope with symptoms. This conclusion has been confirmed by other studies of chronic illness, particularly chronic pain. Emotional stress can be mitigated, but the physical symptoms of CFS are much less likely to respond to cognitive-behavioral methods.

Exercise Intolerance in CFS: Why?

There are three plausible explanations for activity and exercise limitation in CFS:

1. The disabling effects of CFS symptoms

2. Physical deconditioning due to lack of exercise and activity

3. Psychosocial factors

Treadmill studies show that CFS patients terminate treadmill walking before healthy controls due to fatigue buildup. Unfortunately, the physiological reason for this early fatigue is as yet unknown. In the most severely ill, bedridden people with chronic fatigue syndrome, physical deconditioning may be an important factor in activity limitation and easy exhaustion. For such individuals, an intense effort to maintain minimal daily activity is important if they are to avoid physical deconditioning.

However, people with CFS who do several hours a day of paid or unpaid work, or remain at full-time positions that involve several miles of routine walking a day, are probably as active as many healthy individuals, and their level of fitness is probably no worse. I do not think it plausible to attribute their activity limitation to deconditioning. In addition, when a person with CFS can do mild exercise, there is often a feeling of exhilaration *during* the activity, followed by a delayed symptom buildup the next day. This is not the delayed soreness or stiffness anyone might experience, but rather an abnormally severe fatigue that is characteristic of CFS after exercise. If physical deconditioning were the primary cause of symptom flare-ups in CFS, you would expect exhaustion to set in during the exercise, not a day later.

Psychosocial factors refer to emotional and social benefits, or payoffs, that might result from being ill. These payoffs supposedly include avoidance of obligations, and increased attention, love, and support. (A discussion of psychosocial factors in CFS can be found in Step 2.) Psychosocial factors as a comprehensive explanation for activity restrictions have not been verified by any published research. Although the Butler study cited above suggests a psychologically based avoidance of activity, the failure to replicate their findings casts doubt on their conclusions.

My analyses of people with CFS do not support a psychosocial explanation of activity limitation. If you did regular physical exercise prior to the onset of CFS, you're painfully aware of the restrictions that now limit you. You probably still want to exercise, but can only manage a small fraction of the workout you once did. For the individuals with CFS I've seen, there is no psychological payoff in avoiding exercise. If a graduated exercise schedule leading to longer and more vigorous exercise sessions was a partial or total cure for this illness, I think we would have discovered it on our own.

Of course, I cannot speak for other people with CFS who have tried to help themselves with exercise. I base my statement on my own efforts to restore physical exercise of any kind into my schedule. There seems to be a low-level exercise limit that I cannot exceed. I am assuming that others with CFS have reached similar conclusions in their attempts to improve exercise tolerance.

Exercise Alternatives

One jogger with CFS to another: "I start out slow and taper off from there."

One way to gauge the connection between exercise and CFS symptoms is to reduce your exercise or activity level, assuming that you're currently pushing the limit of your endurance. For instance, rather than briskly walking 15 minutes every other day, you might temporarily reduce your workout to 5 minutes of leisurely walking every other day. The lessened exertion may reduce your CFS symptoms and, for some individuals, may promote a less fatigued physical state in general. Starting with this reduced activity level, rebuild your exercise tolerance gradually over several weeks, until you reach and possibly exceed your original levels. Through this retraining process, you may learn some important things about how exercise affects your symptoms.

- Your activity level may indeed have been too high: you may function better, emotionally and physically, doing a lower level of exercise

- A gradual buildup from a very minimal level of activity may allow you to increase your endurance without undue exacerbation of your symptoms

- Your daily physical activity may not be improved by a gradual increase in the level of your activity; but it's probably worth a try to see if this particular method works for you

Alternatively, if your physical activity is almost nil—if you are sitting or lying down nearly all the time—then your risk for a severe depression is much greater. Assuming that you also have an array of cognitive symptoms—including mental fogginess, poor concentration, and memory impairment—the feeling of near-total disability would be a major challenge to anyone's efforts to cope. I would suggest establishing a low-level, daily routine of activity including sitting, walking around the house or out of doors, very light housework, listening to informational tapes or pleasurable music, doing needlework, or easy reading. You can arrange your day into small, manageable segments of activity. If you have not considered antidepressant medication, there are selected low-dosage antidepressants that may reduce your fatigue symptoms and elevate your mood.

There is no blanket prescription for activity and exercise that applies to all people with chronic fatigue syndrome. For most of us who are as active as we can be, increasing activity further is not well-advised. For extremely depressed individuals immobilized by CFS, individually tailored activity schedules and low-dosage antidepressants may be helpful. Most importantly, the activity schedule should be designed to match your own capabilities and preferences. Don't worry about "lost" fitness. If you can maintain a daily routine with some level of physical activity, you greatly decrease your health risk for all causes of mortality. You have about the same risk for life-threatening illness as the most fit.

Step 5

Cope and Hope

Coping Strategies in a Nutshell

There are many things you can do to cope with your CFS symptoms, including:

- Attitudinal adjustments
- Support from yourself and others
- Limiting your activity
- Cultivating spirituality
- Avoiding stress
- Developing new interests, hobbies, or skills
- Reprioritizing goals
- Improving your diet and nutrition
- Self-education
- Panic attacks can be controlled or even eliminated through self-taught, cognitive-behavioral interventions. You can

learn to let go of panicky feelings, rather than dwell on them.

- To reduce your burden of guilt feelings, remind yourself that your worth as a human being does *not* have to be based on how much or how little you're able to accomplish.

- Personal writing can help you resolve past traumas.

Why Do We Need Coping Skills?

In an informative talk given at the 1994 meeting of the American Association for Chronic Fatigue Syndrome, Marjorie J. McKenzie II, M.A., outlined the three main reasons why people with chronic fatigue syndrome need to develop coping skills:

1. To cope with all their symptoms, whether or not they're on the official CDC symptom list

2. To cope with the activity restrictions that the illness places upon their lives, including limits on physical, social, and vocational activities, as well as the internal restrictions they impose on themselves

3. To cope with the disbelief of doctors, insurance companies, family and friends, the media, and even the little voice inside us that says, "Maybe I'm not really sick."

In our study of long-term cases of CFS (Friedberg et al. 1994), we asked people to briefly outline the personal coping strategies they've found most helpful. Table 5 lists the general categories of coping we tallied. The ability to make adjustments in attitude received the most endorsements as a coping skill. Respondents told us, "I stopped comparing myself to others," "I don't waste time worrying about what might have been," "I tell myself this phase will pass, and I dream about a cure," "I remind myself to be in the moment—that's all there is."

Rest and pacing were cited the second most frequently. People said that it helped them to alternate rest and small amounts of activity throughout the day (see Step 4).

Support from oneself and others was also highly rated. This includes reaching out to other people, networking with other patients, congratulating yourself for doing the best you can, and allowing yourself time for self-care, even if others are angry about it.

Limiting your activity, the coping skill that rated fourth on the list, refers to taking assertive self-control to maximize your positive feelings and cut down on symptom-causing activities. The spiritual aspects of coping include prayer, meditation, and yoga. Avoiding stress is somewhat self-explanatory and is the underlying theme of this book.

Table 5. Most Helpful Coping Skills, Based on the Responses of 253 People With CFS

1. Attitudinal adjustments	129
2. Rest and pacing	95
3. Support from yourself and others	95
4. Limiting your activity	90
5. Cultivating your spirituality	77
6. Avoiding stress	73
7. Developing new interests, hobbies, or skills	48
8. Reprioritizing goals	39
9. Improving your diet and nutrition	38
10. Self-education	30

Compiled by Marjorie J. McKenzie II, M.A.

Developing new interests, hobbies, or skills is also an important coping mechanism. This type of activity represents a highly creative way to redirect your behavior in the context of your illness. Pursuit of any of the fine arts—whether music, painting, sculpture, or creative writing—gives you a way to transform your feelings into something beautiful and positive. For a comprehensive list of ideas for creative activities, consult the Pleasant Events Checklist in Appendix B.

For many people in the study, "reprioritizing goals" often involved allowing time for personal matters. Improved diet and nutrition may have a positive effect on your symptoms and your sense of well-being. Self-education about the chronic fatigue syndrome research and advocacy programs will not only keep you informed, but will also generate feelings of self-empowerment.

Ideas for Coping

Coping With Disbelief

Being disbelieved and ignored, it's more difficult to deal with than the illness itself. The word has got to get out to employers and the public that there are illnesses that are disabling but don't have that appearance.

The hardest thing has been the laughter at our expense. Having to pretend to others. To not even tell on a doctor's form that I have CFS for fear he'll dismiss me as a depressed person.

It's so frustrating to feel like death warmed over, but to look good.

Others' disbelief about your illness can cause you to react with anger, frustration, hurt feelings, and guilt—all of which may combine to create tremendous stress. Changing uninformed skepticism about CFS into respect and knowledge may be very difficult. But if we can't convince others about the reality of our illness, we can still find ways within ourselves to reduce the damaging effects of disbelief. Marjorie J. McKenzie II, M.A., suggests that you reduce your sense of isolation by developing a group identity. Get involved with others who understand, accept, or at least tolerate your illness. Develop an underground culture—network with others who have CFS. She also suggests that you can cope with disbelief best by educating yourself: Keep up with the latest research on the illness.

More Coping Suggestions

Despite the overwhelming negatives of this illness, you will probably learn things that strengthen you emotionally. Can you identify anything about this illness that has been helpful to you in some way, whether it is an improved relationship, realizations about your priorities, or even a minor yet constructive change in your life? Any positive element you can define can become the basis for another coping skill that will help you adapt to the illness.

Here's a list of strategies I've used to reduce stress and encourage a more positive outlook:

- Wake up each day and ask yourself, "How am I feeling? What can I do with the energy I have? If I don't have any, in what ways can I rest until my energy returns?" When you do rest, say to yourself, "I need the rest—this is good."

- Practice personal stress management. Learn to identify the body symptoms and signals of excess stress. Identify the triggering situations, such as a particular conversation, person, or activity. Then use self-relaxation (Step 3) and pacing (Step 4) to alleviate your stress.

- Identify personality traits you may have that drive you to pursue activities beyond your energy limits. For instance, many individuals with CFS like to help people. But you can easily exhaust yourself and deplete your energy by helping or "rescuing" others. Recognize that adequate time for yourself is your right and duty. If you don't take care of yourself, you won't have the energy you need to help others.

- Set limits to your social commitments. That's a tough one, because you may risk disapproval, and a consequent loss of friends. Ask yourself if avoiding disapproval is worth the personal price of overexertion and possible collapse. For the friends you do lose, tell yourself that it's their decision rather than your fault or responsibility. Recognize that many friendships are based on unwritten rules, such as "You will be available to me X hours per week, month, etc." Unfortunately, many friendships are contingent on certain behaviors; unconditional friendships are possible, but rare. Recognize that the friendships that endure despite your illness are the most valuable ones.

- Avoid involvements with negative people. The consequences of CFS are bad enough. Trading nothing but horror stories or complaints with others will deplete your limited energies in an unconstructive way. Become sensitive to the differences between networking with other CFS sufferers, and wallowing with them in mutual misery. Your best companions may be people who have CFS, but are still upbeat.

- Seek out positive news and information. Listen to uplifting speakers on subjects that interest you. Decide to avoid negative information that may influence your mood. This may be as simple as not watching the local TV news.

- Find another individual with CFS, and begin to build a rapport between you. Contact each other regularly to express feelings, discuss news, and provide mutual support. In this way, you are not only helping, but you are being helped as well. Reciprocal relationships like this will make social contact less stressful for you.

- If you're involved in any organizations—such as a parents' association, or a community or church group—recognize that you don't have to be the leader or organizer. You can be part of the group to the extent that your energy level allows: your contribution is still important in the context of your role as a participant rather than a leader.

- Keep the word "hope" in your thinking. Currently, there is no cure for CFS. But followup studies of CFS patients have revealed that many people improve and some people do recover, sometimes after two years, five years, or even twenty years (Lapp 1994). There *is* reason for hope. While you are ill, various medications may provide temporary symptom relief. You need not let go of your dreams and goals just because you have CFS. This isn't denial, because you may not always have CFS. It's important to hold onto this possibility. We will tolerate our symptoms but perhaps never accept them. Hope and belief can take root on those days when your symptoms are minimal. Practice visualization and relaxation at these times, as well as when you're feeling really bad.

- Learn the art of total absorption. One person I know spent a morning at the beach watching someone build sand castles. She was so immersed in her observations that this normally unremarkable activity became completely enjoyable and relaxing. Absorption can be achieved by reading a spellbinding novel, listening to an inspirational speaker, being in nature, or even having sex. Absorption in something you enjoy is a powerful coping technique for this illness. You can almost forget about it for long intervals of time.

- For more ideas, look at the personal list below of an individual with CFS. It consolidates many of the suggestions offered in this book into six compelling thoughts about illness-related issues. Also consult the list of "Coping Strategies Gathered From Around the World" in Appendix C, based on the responses of 265 people with CFS. This extensive catalog of ideas is direct, personal, and well-focused on illness issues.

Six CFS Ideas*

1. *Whether or not I can convince someone I have CFS, I will probably wake up sick tomorrow.*

    Often, it seems to me, we are too concerned about convincing others that we are really sick, as if having someone believe us is going to help us directly. Though it is important to have those close to us understand our illness, we should also learn not to care what people who don't matter that much to us think.

2. *Find something that you can do—and then do it.*

    I've found that lowering my short-term standards and goals to a level I am capable of reaching helps quite a bit. Of course, this doesn't mean giving up the long-term goal of health.

3. *Virtually everything we've been through because of our illness, someone else has been through.*

    Everybody experiences much of the same things with our illness, and it's important to realize this. It's often the small things in life (taking out the trash, being able to read, etc.)

---

* *Based on work by Ron Hill.*

that people beat themselves up over the most, and realizing just how many of these small things we share with each other is important.

4. *Despite our illness, we are still more like other people than unalike.*

   It's easy to get into a mode of "all my problems are because of CFS," especially when you are discovering all the ways in which it directly or indirectly affects your life. What is often the case is that "all my problems are affected by my CFS." It's often helpful to realize that many of those problems are problems shared with everybody.

5. *Don't let anyone convince you that psychology, diet, viruses, genetics, etc. are solely responsible for your illness. On the other hand, don't discount the fact that some or all of these may play a role.*

   Whether or not a single virus causes CFS for a particular person, *after* someone is ill, other things like diet, how you react emotionally, allergies, rest, etc. play a role. This is particularly important when it comes to psychology. Since people are always blaming us for our symptoms, we sometimes tend to ignore the emotional part of our life when it could be helpful in dealing with our illness.

6. *There is probably not one thing that will cure me, but there may be value in many different things.*

   It's easy to get into the mode of waiting for the "miracle cure." Whether or not that will ever come is almost irrelevant to how we feel today. Many people report having some improvement in symptoms from different types of therapies, and when you are as sick as CFS people often are, even some improvement can be a lot.

Alleviate Panic Attacks

Among people with CFS, about one person in ten experiences panic attacks. A panic attack is a brief episode of terror or dread accompanied by several of the following symptoms:

- Difficulty breathing

- Heart palpitations

- Dizziness or lightheadedness

- Sweating palms

- Trembling

- Chest pain

- Nausea

- Chills or hot flashes

- Feelings of unreality

- A sense of impending doom that may be focused on a fear of fainting, having a heart attack, going crazy, or losing control

When a panic attack is associated with a particular situation or event, the individual may then avoid that situation, fearing that the panic attack will recur. This is a phobic reaction. Common phobias include fear of enclosed places, such as stores or restaurants, where "escape" may be difficult, or any other situation in which a "trapped" feeling may arise, such as being in crowds, a moving car or bus, or waiting in line. The experience of panic is so overwhelming that it may be hard to believe that you can solve the problem in a fairly straightforward manner.

Panic attacks persist as long as the individual fears subsequent attacks. This fear may be generated by particular situations in which panic attacks have occurred, or by paying attention to bodily sensations that seem to signal an impending attack. The type of beliefs that maintain panic include:

- "What if I have another attack? I might pass out (or have a heart attack or go crazy)."

- "I can't stand the feeling of panic."

- "It would be much too embarrassing to have a panic attack in public."

- "I must analyze each attack to see if something really terrible will happen."

All of these self-statements will sustain fear and fuel further attacks. Panic symptoms create fear. Fear, in turn, generates more symptoms.

The first step in controlling the fear/panic cycle is to prove to yourself that the likelihood is minimal of a heart attack or any other acute medical condition being triggered by a panic attack. The proof is found in the medical literature: *panic attacks do not trigger severe medical problems.* Secondly, recognize that you are insisting on a "no panic" guarantee as a precondition to going somewhere. This belief is an impossible demand: you cannot obtain such a guarantee. When you surrender the idea of the guarantee, then you confront the worst thing that could possibly happen: you will feel very uncomfortable. That's it—the worst. Thirdly, convince yourself that you can tolerate the discomfort. As you give up the notion of guaranteed poise and comfort in any situation, the frequency of panic attacks will decrease. You can also use the relaxation techniques outlined in Step 3 to cope with attacks.

Finally, you need not berate yourself for having panic attacks. They are nothing more than maladaptive habits based on physical and psychological factors. These habits can be changed through cognitive-behavioral interventions and, in some cases, with medication. The coping statements below will help you change the maladaptive habits that may have made you susceptible to panic attacks. As you repeat these statements to yourself, you will begin to internalize the message that improved tolerance of the discomforts of panic will lead to greater feelings of control and a reduced frequency of panic episodes. In most cases, individuals who practice these self-suggestions for only two five-minute periods a day will reduce their panic attacks to a very low level, and perhaps to nothing.

Coping Statements for Panic Attacks *

1. Feelings of panic are distressing, but not dangerous.

2. Feelings are not facts.

3. These feelings will pass: they are temporary.

---

* *Adapted from Weekes (1969).*

4. These feelings seem to be telling me that something terrible will happen; in reality, my body is overreacting to excess adrenaline, nothing more.

5. I will try to accept my feelings, not fight them off. Fighting only creates more tension.

6. I will face my feelings, not run away from them.

7. If others think I'm strange, it's uncomfortable for me; but I can tolerate being looked at or even judged.

Reducing Guilt: The Impossible Dream?

I teach people with CFS to use phrases such as, "Relax, cope, feel better." And it may well work. Your mind begins to release the negative thinking and feelings associated with the illness. But the feeling of guilt does not yield so easily. Why? Guilt is the result of falling far short of our self-image as helpers and givers. After all, who are we if we can't perform these roles? Aren't we bad people? Perhaps, we fear, we've entered the ranks of the sub-humans.

But should we feel guilty? It's obvious that we can't do certain things that are important to us and others. I don't think we can logically fault ourselves, but we do anyway. Guilt alleviation is advantageous, because it removes a negative, useless feeling. Guilt may be a form of self-punishment, but aren't we punished enough with our restrictions? Remove the guilt and we will still continue to do what we can.

The first step in reducing guilt is to recognize that you are rating yourself as a human being based on certain behaviors. The thinking process might go, "As a caregiver, I can accept myself. When I am less of a caregiver, I am less of a human being." But you can prove to yourself how inaccurate this statement is and feel better. Reserve two five-minute periods a day to read and reread the following guilt-reducing statements (based on rational emotive principles, Ellis 1973):

1. I have the right to feel the guilt that I feel but I also recognize its destructive effects.

2. I can rate my behaviors as good or bad, but my behaviors do not define me as a person. If I can't do what I have in the past, this is regrettable and unfortunate—but it does not lessen my worth as a human being.

3. When I'm performing well, I don't then rate myself as a great or totally good person. So why berate myself for those things I can't do now? I can dislike the restriction while still accepting myself.

4. I had more control over my life before the illness. It's unfair to tell myself that I should have that same control now. I don't need the extra pressure. I can learn to control my emotional and behavioral reactions to the illness, but there is no evidence that I should know how to act 100 percent normal with CFS.

5. The illness is most certainly limiting and inconvenient, but I can learn not to think of it as totally devastating. Even many disadvantages do not equal devastation. If I can offer myself any reason to live with this illness, then I am acknowledging hope and optimism, however small.

The Three Stages of Relief From Guilt

As you internalize these ideas, you are likely to feel relief from guilt in three distinct stages:

Stage 1—Skepticism. Your reasoning might be: "I really don't know if I can stay calm, and accept myself, and say, 'Okay, this is me, and I am limited. I won't be able to accomplish as much as I used to, but it's okay if I don't.' I really have a problem with this— I'm not sure I really believe it. If I can't perform, then what am I going to do? I've always judged my worth by my actions."

Stage 2—Belief. As you face the uncertainty of this illness, you can let go of that desperate feeling that you must control yourself as well as you did prior to being ill. You now recognize the burden of feeling guilty—it wastes your energy. You can begin to stop comparing what you did before with what you can do now. You might tell yourself, "Okay, I'm going to let go of who I was. If I can re-cover some part of that, great; if I can't, I'll just focus on what I hope to be able to do, say, a year from now. My goals will be mod-est and attainable."

Stage 3—Internalization. You may not fully achieve this level of conviction, but anyone with CFS can at least approach it. The question-and-answer format below may well correspond to the two sides of yourself: The guilty/blaming self and the rational/tolerant self. Internalization implies a strong belief in the rational self.

Guilt/Worry Statement: What if I can't take care of the house the way I used to, fulfill my work deadlines, etc.? How can I not judge myself harshly?

Rational Response: In the larger scheme of things, it doesn't matter so much if there's something I can't do. As I think this, it relieves me of useless guilt, and I begin to realize how many things I do that are not that important, that are just energy drainers. And if I discover that I have energy for only a few important activities, I will just try to focus on those. I will limit my social commitments. I will not drive myself into the ground anymore. If anything gets done, it gets done. If it doesn't, that's too bad.

If people around you start expecting things that you know you can't deliver, then it's up to you to stop yourself and say, "Look, I can't do this."

One individual with CFS told me how she was walking down stairs one day when someone began talking to her. She responded, "Don't talk to me, because I have to concentrate on going down the steps or else I'm going to fall." If you can express such thoughts to people around you, then you have begun to achieve a strong sense of autonomy and self-control. Rather than thinking, "I'll just put up with this or that situation," you can learn to be more selec-tive. You can avoid unnecessary stress, and feel better both emo-tionally and physically.

Resolving Past Traumas

Dr. Karen Schmaling, a psychologist and CFS researcher at the Uni-versity of Washington in Seattle, studied the psychosocial histories of a small sample of people with the illness and found that a majority of them reported physical or sexual abuse during childhood. In comparison, significantly fewer people who were depressed (without CFS) reported this type of past trauma. If you have a traumatic event in your past that is not fully resolved, I can offer a straightforward technique that may improve your adjustment.

I am not proposing a full treatment for trauma, especially severe trauma. Generally, the more severe the trauma, the more benefit you may receive from psychotherapy. If you are currently in treatment for trauma, please discuss the use of this technique with your therapist or counselor before you try it. The writing technique below may cause a cathartic release of repressed emotion. This may indeed be a healthy event, but the writing technique alone is not a substitute for therapy. Given these precautions, you can decide whether you wish to try the technique of cathartic writing.

Dr. James Pennebaker has published a series of studies (1988) on relieving trauma by detailing the event in writing. Allow yourself a 30-minute writing interval every day for the next four days. Explore your most traumatic, unresolved experience by converting the thoughts and memories into a written account. Unresolved, stressful events from your past would include any incidents that remain prominent in your thinking. Such an incident is still upsetting. You may try to block out the recurring memories. It may disturb your sleep; and it may interfere with your relationships. Prior stressful events that may be associated with ongoing emotional difficulty include physical, sexual, or emotional abuse; death or separation from a loved one; auto accidents; work-related injuries; crime victimization; or natural disasters such as a hurricane, tornado, or earthquake. As you write down the memory, include as much emotional content as you can. Just allow your memories to flow onto the paper.

The writing down of past trauma will produce an emotional release, as well as an autonomic physical release. In prior studies of this phenomenon, improvements in immune function have been noted for people who write down their traumas. Another interesting result is that individuals who wrote down their traumas had fewer visits to health providers than a control group that wrote about ordinary, daily events.

The recording of traumas may work in a manner similar to individual counseling, which also facilitates an emotional release through the discussion of painful events.

Positive Aspects of Religious Belief

Some people with chronic fatigue syndrome ask themselves, "Why is God punishing me?" It may be a struggle for some of us not to believe that this illness wasn't God's will. That is a depressing thought to have about a loving, creative being. But you can learn to change your way of thinking. It's impossible to prove that any-one "deserves" to have this illness. Among the scores of patients with CFS I've seen, there isn't any indication that they have con-ducted their lives in an immoral way, or that they are in any way deserving of such a punishment as this illness. The phrase, "It's God's will," reduces a complicated issue to a cliché that explains little. Whatever your religious belief, there is no logical way to con-nect it with the experience of this illness.

Focus instead on the uplifting aspects of your spiritual beliefs. Prayer gives solace and a feeling of inner-directedness. Reading re-ligious writing can provide inspiration. Attending religious services can reinforce your beliefs in transcendence. If possible, attend a healing mass or service. Some people with CFS have been helped by such rituals.

> I've had CFS for the past 18 months. Although I am not a very religious person, I attended a healing service in which the minister, after a brief but inspirational sermon, asked everyone to stand up and then to fall down. Everyone in the service fell down, including myself. I didn't intend to fall down, it just happened. This is called being "slain in the spirit." I had some sort of epiphany or communication with God, I think. After the service, I felt transformed emotionally and physically. My CFS symptoms were 80 percent gone. The cognitive difficulty was still present,

although to a lesser degree. I don't understand quite
how and why this happened, but I am just glad it did.

I knew this person through therapy sessions. I have not heard
such a miraculous story of healing either before or since. I started
reading religious literature myself, impressed as I was. Your religious belief can be a rich resource whether you experience healing
or not.

Support Groups: Benefit or Burden?

By giving talks to many CFS support groups, I have come away
with my own impression of what makes a support group work for
its participants. The elements of a successful group appear to be a
strong yet empathic leader and an agenda for meetings that emphasizes inspirational speakers who can provide useful information about various aspects of the illness. An effective group leader
will allow time for speaker presentations, questions and answers,
updates on CFS information, and at the end of the meeting, time
for a more personalized exchange about the illness among those
who wish to participate.

Support group meetings are less successful when they become
a forum for exchanging complaints; or, at the other extreme, when
they allow virtually no time for participant input. Because of the
stress that everyone carries with them to these meetings, talking
about symptoms and problems can become a competition to see
who is suffering more. If you encounter such a gathering, speak to
the group leader about restructuring meetings as recommended
above. Such positive changes will probably increase group mem-
bership and make the meetings more helpful for everyone involved.

Summing Up

The following quote from a person with a long-term case of CFS
reflects his long period of evolution and adjustment to the illness.

This individual has clearly claimed priority for his health and well-being:

> Don't take anything less than the best treatment from a doctor. If he or she can't treat your symptoms, teach them. If they won't be taught, sue them! Don't let the medical profession, Social Security, or your insurance company give you anything but full cooperation and kindness. CFS is not the end of the world. It may be almost dead last, but it's not the end. Learn about it, let it teach you, stay ahead of the game, be reasonable, but be firm.

Step 6

Induce a Positive Mood, Minimize Setbacks

Coping Strategies in a Nutshell

- Everyone has daily fluctuations in their mood and energy levels, with peak times when they feel good and perform optimally. It's especially important for people with CFS to become aware of when these peak times occur, and to learn to make the most of them.

- High levels of emotional stress can trigger a relapse of symptoms. Learning to minimize stress—or to back away from it—can help you nurture your good moods and make them last as long as possible.

- A positive outlook can actually reduce the severity of symptoms. You can learn the technique of pleasant mood induction to generate and sustain a positive mood.

- Focusing on humor and laughter can help sustain your good moods. Laughter has health benefits as well.

- A good mood can quickly erode as you turn your attention to stressful daily activities. Learning to identify the early signs of mood lowering will help you shake off an emerging bad mood before it envelops you.

People with chronic fatigue syndrome, despite their reduced energy levels, still retain a regular daily fluctuation in their energy patterns. There are times during the day, especially in the late morning hours, when both your physical and mental energy levels are higher. These peak energy times are associated with positive feelings. A recent study headed by Dr. C. Wood (1992) found daily fluctuations in energy and positive mood in CFS to be similar to those found in healthy adults, albeit at a lower level. Since all of Dr. Wood's subjects, healthy or ill, reported similar daily patterns, elevated moods and higher energy levels may be part of a daily biological pattern we all have. People with CFS are especially well-advised to become aware of their peak times.

Your capacity to experience and enjoy daily periods of higher energy and uplifted mood will be affected by emotional stress—the third most common relapse trigger for people with CFS, after ordinary physical exertion and exercise (Friedberg et al. 1994). (Of course, any of the relapse triggers listed in Table 6 can deplete our precious feelings of vigor and vitality.) As you learn to control negative emotional reactions to daily stressors, you can allow what positive mood and energy you do have to fully express itself. Tap into this reservoir of good feeling at your peak times and enjoy it fully.

The causes of setbacks and relapses in CFS have only recently been addressed in the research literature. An ongoing study out of southern Florida conducted by Dr. Michael Antoni and his colleagues (Lutgendorf et al. in press) looked at relapse predictors in CFS during Hurricane Andrew, a devastating storm that destroyed thousands of homes and left 75,000 people homeless. In their sample of individuals with CFS who were exposed to the full force of the hurricane, about 40 percent of them relapsed into states of extreme fatigue, higher symptom levels, and increased work disability. The strongest predictor of relapse was high levels of emotional stress. This means that elevated levels of anxiety and depression *before* the hurricane predicted higher levels of relapse. Interestingly, emotional distress was more important than material loss in predicting relapse. This may be somewhat surprising, given that the hurricane had broad-ranging effects, including financial and material losses, as well as death and injury. Of course, severe disruption of social, family, and work routines occurred as well. The authors

Table 6. Relapse Triggers Rated
by Individuals With CFS

Relapse Trigger	CFS Respondents (N=300)
Physical stress (doing too much)	97%
Exercise	85%
Emotional stress (upsets)	80%
Other infections	75%
Emotional trauma	65%
Chemical exposure/ air pollutants	56%
Physical trauma	60%
Humid weather	57%
Allergens	56%
Hot weather	47%
Barometric pressure	45%
Certain foods	43%
Cold weather	41%
Medications	32%
Vaccinations/ immunizations	25%
Pregnancy	13%
Birth control pills/ estrogen supplements	9%

Friedberg et al. (1994)

of the study found that a tendency to cope with CFS through denial of the illness, and "giving up" behavior (reducing coping behavior), was also correlated with relapse. Denial often involves a rejection of a CFS diagnosis, and forceful attempts to avoid thinking about the stress and impairment brought about by the illness.

On the other hand, an optimistic coping style was associated with resistance to relapse and improved levels of Interleukin 4, a chemical messenger of the immune system associated with CFS-like symptoms. Finally, greater levels of social support also were predictive of a lower incidence of relapse.

Of course, normal, healthy adults in the hurricane area suffered physical and emotional stress as well. People with CFS have an increased vulnerability to stressful events that may worsen their symptoms, as well as produce negative emotional outcomes. If we can learn to harness our positive emotional resources, then we will be better able to buffer the effects of stressful life events, and better protect ourselves.

Bearing in mind the findings of Dr. Antoni's research group, it would seem that the steps in this book devoted to strengthening your coping abilities and reducing stress will have the added benefit of helping you minimize your susceptibility to relapses.

Positive Mood as a Symptom Reducer

Peak Experiences

I had been dragging for a couple of weeks. The fatigue was a predominant feature of my daily moods; my sleep was disturbed. This was in late October to early November of '93. As Election Day approached, I became more interested in local political races, and felt absolutely committed to two local candidates. When both of them won stunning upset victories by only slight margins, I revelled in those post-election moments. My mood soared. For the next several days, I felt extremely positive, optimistic, and significantly less fatigued.

I also negotiated a favorable change in my part-time working hours, which further bolstered my mood. My sleep, although not particularly restful, did not weigh on my mind, nor was it a focus of my negative attention. Clearly I was reinforced by an unusually positive series of events. The part that's somewhat surprising is that my fatigue became much less severe and I felt more capable and functional. On the other hand, I'm in a moderately good mood much of the time, yet I don't get such obvious benefits to my fatigue levels.

The above narrative illustrates the powerful mind/body connection in chronic fatigue syndrome. I am not claiming that positive experiences will cure CFS, only that they can significantly diminish its impact. Your ability to create peak experiences may well influence how functional you can be, and how good you can feel. Pleasant mood induction involves either imagining or participating in an activity that, based on prior experience, will uplift your mood and create a positive or euphoric emotional state. According to recent experimental research (Brown et al. 1993), positive mood induction is highly effective in producing elation with healthy changes in stress hormones. Also, pleasant mood induction generates feelings of increased energy or vigor, reduces anger, and improves pain tolerance. These emotional benefits can diffuse the persistent stress of the illness.

Generating peak experiences and sustaining a positive mood is, of course, more difficult when you're ill. However, a simple focusing exercise will allow you to create a repertoire of modest yet uplifting activities.

First, make a list of positive current events in your life. Be inclusive. Major and even minor events are all highly significant: a good movie, a captivating speaker, an intimate moment with your spouse or close friend. Include the little pleasures: taking a bath, reading an absorbing novel, enjoying a positive interaction with your children. If you need help in generating the list, think of events in the past that you enjoyed and could do now, or consult the Pleasant Events Checklist in Appendix B, which contains a list of 300 positive experiences. Write down the items that you would enjoy doing, then select 5 to 10 of your choices and schedule them for the coming week. If your ability to experience a positive mood has been compromised by your illness, this exercise may be an important first step toward freeing yourself to experience pleasure again.

To summarize, the benefits of mood induction will allow you to

- Divert your attention from symptoms
- Replace negative feelings with positive ones
- Lessen fatigue symptoms
- Break out of the fatigue-stress cycle that intensifies fatigue and discouragement (see Step 1)

Humorous Experiences

I attended a professional conference on humor and creativity which focused on integrating humor and laughter into your personal and professional life. I was so uplifted by that conference that I literally forgot about my fatigue—which is something that doesn't happen very often. It was as if it wasn't there.

Clearly I wasn't cured of my fatigue. I don't believe that laughter is a cure; but it was so refreshing and completely diverting to be absorbed in that kind of activity that I sustained the feeling for about a week. I was so impressed that I could have that kind of mental power over my fatigue.

Humor and laughter can be powerful distractions from the stress of our illness (Cousins 1984). A humorous diversion can allow us to "separate" ourselves from fatigue and stress. Laughter stimulates the production of endorphins, our bodies' natural pain killers. Recent research on laughter (Berk et al. 1989; Klein 1989) shows that laughter can enhance immune function, counteract depression, and even substitute, to some extent, for aerobic exercise. Laughter increases your heart rate and respiration, causes huffing and puffing, and gives facial and stomach muscles a workout. Twenty seconds of laughter can double your heart rate for three to five minutes, and is the equivalent of three minutes of strenuous rowing. Laughter is also a natural tension reducer; it produces relaxation for up to 45 minutes afterwards. With humor, we can confront personal problems in a more relaxed and creative state of mind and body.

Laughter *is* good for your health. But how many of us even approach even ten minutes of hearty laughter in the course of a day?

The health benefits of humor can be achieved with just a few minutes of laughter every day. How much time do you spend laughing every day? Ten minutes, one minute, less? If you feel that your ability to appreciate humor has become limited, compose a list of 10 things that ordinarily make you laugh. After completing the list, note by each item how long it has been since you have laughed in response to that particular event. If you can't recall several experiences that have made you laugh recently, think about how you might arrange your schedule to make your life more conducive to laughter.

You don't have to go to a comedy club or watch a funny movie to laugh. You can discover the humor and fun in everyday, ordinary events (Goodman 1988). Things that often don't seem so funny—like the stressors that surround you—often have humorous elements. You can redefine things that appear to be negative and find something humorous in them. Sometimes, at the most unlikely moments, when you feel completely bereft of energy, you can identify something funny. When everything seems to go wrong an opportunity for a humorous take on things is created.

Try one of these suggestions to develop your humor resources:

- Buy books with humorous stories, quotes, or jokes, and identify some that have special meaning for you.

- Put something humorous in your office that also makes a point. One company owner had a life-size picture of her infant grandson with his toe in his mouth, captioned, "Don't let our customers catch you this way!"

- Take a humor break at least once a day.

- Read the comics and save the ones that make you laugh.

- Play cassette tapes of comedy routines while you're driving or doing chores at home. Bill Cosby's routines are particularly irresistible.

- Identify any funny stories or funny things your children have said or done, or times when humor "saved the day" in your family. Describe one or two of these to a friend.

- Go to a playground and watch kids playing. Toddlers can be especially humorous in their interactions.

- Ask friends to share their funniest stories with you. Collect these, and share them with others.

If these suggestions stimulate your interest in nurturing laughter, define what issues or areas of your family life could use some lightening up. For instance, identify one of your pet peeves that might be alleviated with humor.

Another question to ask yourself is, when have you laughed so hard that your mood was uplifted for several hours? I'll offer a personal example:

At age 16, I attended a recital hosted by my sister's piano teacher for all her students. The teacher paraded each of her students onto the stage to play or sing various pieces. One kid was playing a march, which seemed to be going well until he made a mistake in about the middle of the piece. Rather than continuing past it, he kept repeating that measure over and over and over again, trying to get it right. It was like hearing a broken record, but not being able to stop it. As members of the audience, we weren't supposed to laugh; but I started to feel tightness in my stomach from suppressing my laughter. With no time to recover from the previous kid's performance, a girl about 16 years old appeared on the stage to sing Moon River; but her voice was cracking all over the place. Of course you can't laugh, because these kids are very sensitive, and all the proud parents were there, too. I would describe the visceral experience of sitting in that audience as "splitting a gut." After the recital, I must have laughed hard for 10 minutes. It took another hour to calm down.

Can you remember any occasions when you laughed so hard that you felt you were going to lose control of your bladder? Write down two or three personal examples. Read them over once or twice a week to alleviate stress.

As a daily activity, try to revive a funny memory, or look for the ironies and humorous elements in everyday activities. You may have to practice a bit to restore the lighthearted feelings that may have come more easily to you in the past. As much as everyone likes to laugh and have fun, it's more difficult to recapture that lightness when you're facing the problems brought about by a chronic illness.

How To Optimize a Positive, Energetic Mood

Regardless of what event is associated with a good mood, *you* created that good mood through your own thinking. An optimistic, energetic outlook inspired by something external may last from a few hours to a couple of days. Unfortunately, uplifting events just don't occur often enough to sustain an energy-creating mood all the time. So it's important to not just depend on external events to bring you good cheer: you want to learn to nurture your own good moods, and halt the slide into hopelessness, low energy, and depression. Here's a continuation of the story about the person with CFS who felt uplifted by his local election outcome and the improved conditions at his job:

> About a day and a half after the good election news and my successful job negotiation, I was making a long and exhausting series of phone calls. I started to realize that my buoyant mood was eroding quickly, being consumed by fatigue—that abnormal, depressing sort of fatigue that all who have CFS are well aware of. But rather than succumb to the emerging fatigue and malaise, I applied some new ideas to maintain at least part of my positive mood. First, I told myself I

don't have to allow this good feeling to disappear. I became aware of the subtle self-messages, such as, "I'm tired again, there's nothing I can do, this just means more struggle with my fatigue." I challenged these statements by saying, "I don't have to succumb to this! I don't have to passively observe the return of full-blown fatigue. I can change my activities now to something that won't lead to a crash. I can practice my relaxation techniques; I can divert myself with something positive. And I *don't* have to be a slave to my daily obligations at this moment, not if it means feeling exhausted and depleted again."

Become aware of the ways in which a positive mood can rapidly deteriorate. You can learn to nurture an optimistic outlook, and function under its influence, for a much longer time than you may realize. Of course, attention to your thoughts and your mood is essential to success. At any one moment, it may feel easier to do nothing and just allow yourself to surrender a positive feeling. Convince yourself that refocusing your attention is worth the effort.

The following suggestions may help you halt the slide from a positive mood into lethargy:

- Watch for the early signs of mood deterioration and the possible reasons behind it: a shift to negative thinking, a change in behavior to activities or responsibilities that are burdensome, or an unpleasant interaction with other people.

- At the earliest opportunity, choose to shift away from the mood-breaking activity.

- To redirect your attention in a positive way, begin with the *re-lax* phrase (Step 3), or simply take a breather in a way that is pleasing to you. This may only require a minute or two.

- If you return to the original activity that compromised your mood, do it differently—perhaps more slowly, perhaps with more patience. Alternatively, you might want to reschedule it for another time when there's less chance it will get you down.

Step 7

Optimize Emotional Support

Coping Strategies in a Nutshell

- Too much or too little support from your partner may affect both your functioning and stress level. An overprotective partner who does most things for you and tries to shield you from every stress may reduce your feelings of autonomy and self-control. On the other hand, an unsupportive partner may increase your feelings of stress and depression. Talk with your partner—and a marriage counselor, if necessary—to determine your optimum level of support.

- Learn to make the distinction between talking about your emotions and talking about your symptoms. The first kind of talking is beneficial when expressed to a receptive partner or friend. But be careful about finding the appropriate forum for a minute discussion of your symptoms. Discuss symptoms with your doctor, your counselor, and other people who have CFS. However, dwelling too much on your symptoms with your partner or a friend will just exhaust both of you. For a reality check, ask your partner or close friend how you talk about your illness.

- Understand that your partner's reactions and emotions surrounding your illness need to be expressed just as much as yours do. Encourage your partner to express his or her specific concerns. Work together to find compromises so that both of you can get your needs met in the relationship.

Partner Support—How Much Is Enough?

Providing assistance reflects love and caring, but also indicates the dependence and neediness of the recipient. Thus, providing care for someone can be supportive and caring, but can also become controlling and overprotective. Recently emerging literature on partner support in chronic illness suggests that there is an optimal level of support that will best help people who are chronically ill. The results of this research probably apply to people with CFS as well. The difficulty is in defining an optimal level of support: so much depends on the individuals involved, their relationship, and the particular situation.

One way to assess the social support systems of people with CFS, based on in-depth interviews, was developed by Dr. Colette Ray (1992) of Brunel University in England. She devised a 23-item measure that is very sensitive to interpersonal issues in CFS. Take a moment to complete Dr. Ray's inventory, which I've reproduced below. Identify the questions that seem most relevant to your social support situation. For instance, do the answers to particular questions reveal too much or too little support in your life? Do these imbalances influence your mood and, perhaps, your feelings about yourself? It might help to discuss these particular items and concerns with your partner or another close family member or friend.

Social Support Scale

Think of the people in your life who are important to you. The questions below refer to feelings that you might have about them, and the ways in which they respond to you.

Circle one number for each item to indicate the extent to which each description applies. If you want to, you can make a photocopy of the Social Support Scale and fill it out for each significant helper in your life.

Your answer choices are:

1. **Never**
2. **Almost never**

3. Sometimes
4. Quite often
5. Very often
6. Always

1. Can you lean on and turn to them when things are difficult?   1   2   3   4   5   6

2. Can you get a good feeling about yourself from them?   1   2   3   4   5   6

3. Do they put pressure on you to do things?   1   2   3   4   5   6

4. Do they take over your chores when you feel ill?   1   2   3   4   5   6

5. Do they express concern about how you are?   1   2   3   4   5   6

6. Do they misunderstand the way you think and feel about things?   1   2   3   4   5   6

7. Can you trust them, talk frankly, and share your feelings with them?   1   2   3   4   5   6

8. Can you get practical help from them?   1   2   3   4   5   6

9. Do they argue with you about things?   1   2   3   4   5   6

10. Do you feel that they are there when you need them?   1   2   3   4   5   6

11. Do they press you to say that you're feeling better when you're ill?   1   2   3   4   5   6

12. Do they listen when you want to confide about things that are important to you?   1   2   3   4   5   6

13. Do they express irritation with you?   1   2   3   4   5   6

14. Do they accept you as you are, including your failings as well as your stronger points?	1	2	3	4	5	6
15. Do they help out when things need to be done?	1	2	3	4	5	6
16. Do they show you affection?	1	2	3	4	5	6
17. Do they make helpful suggestions about what you should do?	1	2	3	4	5	6
18. Are they critical of the way you respond to illness?	1	2	3	4	5	6
19. Do they do things that conflict with your own sense of what should be done?	1	2	3	4	5	6
20. Do they give you useful advice when you want it?	1	2	3	4	5	6
21. Do they express frustration with you?	1	2	3	4	5	6
22. Do they treat you with respect?	1	2	3	4	5	6
23. Do they disagree with you about what is best for you to do?	1	2	3	4	5	6

Reproduced with permission of author and publisher from:
Ray, C. Positive and negative social support in a chronic illness. *Psychological Reports*, 1992, 71, 977-978. © Psychological Reports 1992

Can Emotional Support Be Bad?

A recent study by Dr. Karen Schmaling on CFS and family reactions to it poses some interesting questions that you may want to ask yourself. The study compared people with CFS who were in good, supportive marriages, versus those who were in unhappy, unsupportive marriages. The findings suggested that people in supportive relationships spent more time lying down than the people in unsupportive relationships. One implication is that a supportive spouse may allow you more time to rest while he or she helps with unfinished chores. The danger of that partner support is that you do less and less rather than push yourself to do as much as you possibly can. In this light, a supportive relationship may encourage helplessness, because others do what you might do for yourself if you weren't being so expertly nurtured.

Other evidence from this marital study highlights the beneficial effect of spousal support. Dr. Schmaling compared stress and depression levels in the satisfying relationships versus the unsatisfying ones. As might be expected, the individuals in satisfying relationships were less stressed and pressured. In unsupportive relationships, the people with chronic fatigue syndrome were more pressured and stressed. The result? They lay down less and were more likely to do work. (In fairness to Dr. Schmaling's study, I am interpreting her data differently than she did.) In short, a healthy relationship may afford you time to rest and recover your energy so you can complete some tasks without risking collapse. An unsupportive spouse may expect more work from you, increasing the risk of symptom flare-ups and setbacks.

With CFS, we do not want to feel any more debilitated than we already are. We prefer to participate in our usual activities as much as possible, and hope that our partner will take over at the times we need to rest and recover. An optimal level of practical and emotional support means that our partner provides the level of support we want—no more, no less. Too much support, especially when your disability is severe, will cause distress, because it makes you feel helpless and incapable. Current research (Spacapan and Oskamp 1992) suggests that chronically ill adults who are overprotected by family caregivers cope less successfully with their disease and have lower feelings of control. Overprotectiveness in chronic illness has been associated with greater levels of depression as well. On the other hand, with too little support our fatigue is more likely to overwhelm us and cause additional stress.

How do we define overprotectiveness? It may mean that your partner is doing too much for you, however well intentioned. This creates a helpless, out-of-control feeling in the person who's ill. A partner who is actually resentful about his or her caregiving role may come across as overprotective. Spacapan and Oskamp, in a 1992 study, suggest that those people who shield their ill partners from upsetting news or difficult decisions may also trigger feelings of being overprotected. The best way to clarify such issues is to get them out into the open. Make sure that your partner has the opportunity to express his or her feelings—and take care to be a good listener.

If you feel overprotected, attempt to analyze the basis of your feelings. Does your partner

1. Resent you?

2. Buffer upsetting information before telling you?

3. Attempt to control you?

4. Derive satisfaction from taking care of you?

The next step is to have a frank discussion with your partner to foster insight into his or her overprotective behaviors. Such a conversation, if carried out with tact and sensitivity, can lead to a mutually agreeable plan to keep the assistance at an optimum level.

Open communication will reduce resentment, and help resolve conflict. For instance, if you do not want your partner to shield you from negative information and feelings, an assertive statement to that effect may help to discourage your partner's overprotective inclinations. Couples who are able to freely express their feelings and emotions about the illness and its consequences have higher levels of marital satisfaction. Spouses of ill partners also have better emotional outcomes if they consider their partners as confidants. Communicate to your partner that he or she doesn't have to solve your problems. Just listening, without judgment, is all that is necessary.

> Couples who worked collaboratively, despite a chronic illness, used sentimental types of interaction, such as giving affection, saying please and thank you, giving compliments, telling the other how much what has been done is appreciated, and doing special little things for the other. (Spacapan and Oskamp 1992, pg. 142)

It's important to distinguish between two different types of discussions about your illness: feelings and reactions about the illness and its consequences, and talk that is focused on a discussion of your symptoms.

You need someone to talk to about your emotions surrounding CFS; so does your partner. A partner who is good at listening can allow you to discharge stressful feelings, feel more relaxed, and even provide a temporary mood boost. Talking about symptoms may be another matter. It's important to find an appropriate forum for detailing CFS symptoms. A CFS-knowledgeable professional or person with CFS can best understand your symptoms. No partner can replace an empathic physician, therapist, or counselor; and no partner can give you the same kind of listening you can get from someone else with CFS.

The danger is that talking too often about symptoms can encourage you to dwell on them in an unhealthy manner. Talking continually about your symptoms can alienate your partner. Also, dwelling on symptoms is more likely to trigger your own feelings of depression. A recent study of lupus, a fatiguing neurological illness, appeared to confirm this distinction between expressing emotions and talking about symptoms. Try to become aware of the content of what you say to your partner; and ask for feedback. What are his or her perceptions about the ways you talk about your illness?

Caregivers Need Support Too

Your spouse or significant other has had to make wrenching adjustments to your illness. He or she may experience the same denial, anger, and even depression that you have in dealing with CFS. It's important that you reserve time with your partner to address his or her personal reactions to the changes that have occurred in your relationship. Try to choose times when you have the emotional energy to sustain such a discussion; or, if a face-to-face encounter is too exhausting, lighten up the pressure by writing each other little notes on the same notepad and passing it back and forth.

Your partner has the same right to all of the negative emotional reactions you have to the illness. Allowing him or her to be heard may solve no practical problem, but it will engender an important emotional release. For instance, your partner may say that he or she is annoyed or even angry that you cannot do certain things. Rather than think of yourself as a convicted felon, understand that your partner is deprived of some level of care and companionship because of your illness. That is not your fault; nor is it your responsibility to immediately (or magically) restore what has been lost. But at least your partner has had the chance to unburden some negative feelings.

Find out what losses have been most significant to your partner. These might include companionship, childcare, housework, sex, going out, and any number of other activities. Ask your partner to make up a list of the most-missed things, and then think about how you can both juggle your priorities to make some changes. If your partner needs more hugs from you, and more "down time" together, maybe you can both find time by relaxing your standards for housekeeping. Look for ways to nurture your life together, so that you're not simply working on opposite shifts. Talk to a marriage counselor if you think you'd be better able to work out adjustments with the help of a competent, sympathetic third party.

Step 8

Design a Healthy Environment

Coping Strategies in a Nutshell

- Find out what local resources are available for disabled people in your area, even if you don't usually label yourself as "disabled." An independent living center (ILC) may offer services that would be useful to you. Look in your telephone directory under Social Services, call the State Vocational Rehabilitation Agency, or contact Independent Research Utilization, 2323 South Shepherd, Suite 1000, Houston, TX 77019, (713) 520-0232.

- Create sanctuary wherever you can find it: in time alone, in nature, on vacation, or in a new home more conducive to recovery.

- To the extent feasible, purge your home environment of toxic chemicals and allergens.

- Organize your household so that you can be as productive and self-sufficient as possible, given the limitations imposed by your illness.

Finding Sanctuary

Selected environments can help people heal by providing them sanctuary from the stressors and conflicts of everyday life. On the other hand, "toxic" environments can interfere with the body's efforts to resist disease. The following passage was written in 1942, and yet its suggestions about changing your surroundings could be applied to the stressors we encounter with CFS.

> In normal primitive life, men commonly had periods of stimulated living, alternated with periods of quiet vegetating. The nervous and physiological reserves consumed during periods of stress were renewed during quiet periods. This was the general condition of primitive village life. Under city influences, especially under modern conditions of constant overstimulation, there is small opportunity for renewing these reserves. There is reason to believe that periods of intense urban life may consume the reserve of human energies to such a degree as to bring about general decadence. Can development of small community living add to its stimulus and interest and yet give opportunity for renewing these reserves and might such an achievement be a major factor in lengthening the period of vital life of a people? (Morgan 1942)

Our CFS symptoms leave us overwhelmingly tired. In an effort to conserve energy, particularly during the worst phases, many people with chronic fatigue syndrome isolate themselves from friends, family, and work. Difficulties maintaining employment can drain financial resources, and may force people with this illness to seek less expensive housing. Feeling ill and isolated, and lacking resources, it is not surprising that many CFS-affected people experience an escalating spiral of negative emotional and physical stressors. Too often, a one-hour monthly support group is all the help that is available.

Dr. Leonard Jason (1993) has proposed the development of healthy settings for people with chronic fatigue syndrome that would involve ongoing supportive care and fellowship: where in-

dividuals could feel accepted and appreciated, and would have op-
portunities to begin re-developing physical capacities that have
withered. Although few ideal settings like this exist, incorporation
of more environmental strategies into comprehensive care for CFS-
affected people seems to be especially warranted. Perhaps such settings would allow people with the illness to strengthen their
immune systems through a variety of medical, nutritional, and environmental interventions. Other non-afflicted people might volunteer as aides in such settings.

A supportive milieu for disabled individuals *is* currently available on an outpatient basis. An independent living center (ILC)
offers a wide variety of services to people with all types of disabilities. Hundreds of ILCs located around the country offer information and referrals. They provide peer counseling to examine and
solve practical problems, and advocacy to obtain support services
and help people with disabilities live more independently.

To locate an ILC in your community, look in your local telephone directory under Social Services; call the main office of the
State Vocational Rehabilitation Agency; or contact Independent Research Utilization, 2323 South Shepherd, Suite 1000, Houston, TX
77019, (713) 520-0232.

In addition to an ILC, think about finding personal sanctuary
in other supportive or, at least, non-stressful environments. Here
are some suggestions:

- Take yourself regularly to a personally non-stressful or uplifting environment. This could mean driving to a local
  park by yourself to allow restful contemplation without in-
  terruption, or renting a funny videotape and spending the
  afternoon in bed with yourself, enjoying a good laugh.

- If you have the financial resources, you may benefit from
  extended vacations to low-stress, positive environments
  where you can still maintain a sense of autonomy and
  modest accomplishment.

- Consider moving. It sounds radical, but certain environments are better suited than others for symptom reduction
  and stress control. Because CFS may be partly generated
  by toxic substances or allergens in the environment, you

may feel better in geographic locations where these toxins are not so prevalent. The list of relapse triggers in Step 6 shows that many individuals with CFS rate chemical exposure, allergens, and specific types of weather conditions (such as humid or hot weather) as important relapse factors. A geographic move can also shield you from stress generated by friends, neighbors, and even family. Be sure to consider carefully before making any permanent move that will make you more socially isolated or deprive you of your usual sources of support.

All of the above strategies may help protect you from the ravages of immune-depressing chemicals and stress. A surge in positive emotions may enhance recovery of formerly impaired immune functions. A new sense of hope and optimism may allow healing to take place.

Design a Healthy Home Environment

Because CFS symptoms may be generated in part by toxic substances or allergens in the home where you spend much of your day, it may be well worth your while to try to purge your home of these harmful materials. Of course, ordinary physical exertion, emotional stress, and family conflict can exacerbate your symptoms as easily as allergenic substances and low-level toxic exposure. It may take some detective work on your part to separate these potential causes of symptom flareups.

If you're uncertain about the extent of your sensitivities to substances in your environment, you can undertake a brief experiment that may yield symptom improvements (Rogers 1986). Your bedroom, where you spend much of your time, is a natural laboratory for identifying symptom-producing substances. Inhalants such as house dust and molds are the most common indoor allergenic materials. Because you probably spend a lot of time in your bed, purging your bed of allergens is an important first step. Encase your pillows, mattress, and boxspring with vinyl coverings. Change your pillowcases daily, and the bedding once a week. Remove all carpeting and rugs, which are dust collectors, and all wall hangings, and vacuum regularly under the bed. Keep all clothing in a closed closet or chest of drawers. Purchase an ionizing air filter. These usually cost less than $50, and produce health-promoting negative ions, as well as clearing dust and dirt out of the air.

Mold growth is more likely to occur in cool, damp environments. If you are mold-sensitive, consider using a dehumidifier in any room where you spend time, especially a basement area during warmer weather. Wash the walls with a disinfectant to eliminate mold growth in rooms that tend to get damp and humid.

I used to experience a profound mental fogginess in the morning that lasted up to an hour after I awoke. Realizing that I'm sensitive to dust and mold, I took steps to reduce these irritants from my environment. My cleanup efforts eliminated the foggy feelings almost immediately.

If such avoidance techniques cause your symptoms to lessen, you may wish to consider allergy testing and treatment to bolster your defenses against environmental allergies.

If you suspect chemical sensitivities, learn to make your environment as pollution-free as possible. The strip-down bedroom techniques will also reduce your exposure to any synthetic chemicals in your bedding materials. Use cotton sheets if you can afford them. Avoid all pesticide use in and outside of your home. If you live in a house or apartment with wall-to-wall carpeting or a lot of plastic or particleboard, try to keep a flow of fresh air through your rooms—especially in the room where you sleep. Don't have your clothes dry-cleaned, if you can avoid this, as the solvents used also emit low-level toxic fumes. If you must dry-clean, hang the clothes outside (or away from your bedroom) for several days before wearing them. Beware of the chemicals in cleaning products and cosmetics. Look for labels that specify that a product is "environmentally safe." What's safe for the environment will be safest for you, too. Avoid cigarette smoke, gasoline fumes, and any other noxious emissions that may trigger a relapse of your symptoms. Try to eat organically grown fruits and vegetables if these are available where you live. Avoid processed foods, food coloring, and chemical additives. Many people believe that supplements of naturally derived Vitamin E and beta carotene (pro-Vitamin A) can help your body purge itself of pollutants. There are books available in the library that can help you identify common household and environmental pollutants. Experiment with these relatively simple measures to see if they relieve any of your symptoms.

Organize at Home

Your home environment can be structured to maximize your feelings of control and self-sufficiency. Judy Basso has written a self-help pamphlet for the National Chronic Fatigue Syndrome and Fibromyalgia Association, 3521 Broadway, Suite 222, Kansas City, MO 64111, (816) 931-4777. She makes the following useful suggestions:

- Consolidate and simplify tasks. Typing uses less energy than writing. When cooking, double the quantity and freeze part for later.

- Organize your household by keeping all the equipment necessary for one task together in one area.

- Sit down whenever possible to conserve energy. Having a high stool to use at the kitchen counter can reduce fatigue and pain.

- Divide more difficult tasks into smaller steps, and take frequent breaks. Try to think of jobs that are compatible with your lowest energy level, such as writing a note to someone special, paying a bill, working on needlecrafts, or putting some pictures in a photo album. Work on these when you have very little stamina. You'll feel good knowing that you were able to complete a project in spite of your limitations.

Step 9

Improve Your Memory

Coping Strategies in a Nutshell

- Use memory aids to help you: write things down in a date-book or on stick-on notes posted around the house. Use visualization both to fix things in your memory and to re-cover them. "Sing" or read information out loud to help your brain record it.

- Keep distractions to a minimum when you need to do any-thing requiring concentration. Work in a quiet room. Prac-tice your breathing and relaxation exercises to clear your mind of internal distractions.*

- Develop the habit of forming mental pictures, and make them as distinct as possible. Create mental associations when you first encounter information you want to remem-ber later on.

---

* Bad moods, depression, and anxiety will also make it harder for you to concen-trate or remember things clearly.

- Be selective in what you try to remember. People who can remember everything are the exception rather than the norm. Be tolerant of yourself when you can't remember something or can't find the right words.

How CFS Affects Memory

Several neuropsychological studies have now been published documenting selective cognitive impairments in CFS patients. To date, the most consistent cognitive deficits have been found on measures of sustained attention. A study done by Drs. John DeLuca, Susan Johnson, and Ben Natelson have confirmed that the ability of people with CFS to shift from one mental task to another, and then return to the original, is significantly disrupted. These findings may well correspond to what people with chronic fatigue syndrome know intuitively. Our train of thought, our ability to think in a logical fashion, can be easily disrupted if we are even momentarily distracted by something else. How often have you gone from one room to another in your house for a particular reason, only to forget why you made the trip? Significantly, the cognitive research findings show that test performance was not related to severity of depressive symptoms, which might have been an alternative explanation for the deficits.

In another study by Dr. Lauren Krupp, myself, and colleagues (1994), about one in four CFS subjects showed difficulty on another test of attention, a visuo-motor tracking task. In the real world, such deficits may be expressed as difficulty in finding your way (in other words, keeping on track) when traveling from one place to another.

Overall, the neuropsychological findings have not confirmed major deficits in memory, which is surprising, given how much anecdotal evidence there is that our memories have been affected. Perhaps one reason for this lack of confirmation in the research is that the standard tests measure gross cognitive abnormalities (such as those found in traumatic brain injury), and may not be sensitive to the lesser degree of memory impairment experienced by people with CFS. This may explain why the attention span studies did show cognitive impairments in CFS: the specific attention measures used were quite sensitive to difficulties in focusing on multiple tasks.

Obviously, more research needs to be done in this area of inquiry. But even if "science" doesn't tell us that we need to work on improving our memories, our own experience points us in that direction.

Memory Boosting Techniques

The first thing to recognize with impairments in memory, attention, and concentration is that these symptoms seem to be an inherent part of CFS. Even if you're depressed about the illness, depression alone does not create these difficulties, and you can't make them disappear simply by trying harder. However, you can use the personal skills you do have to compensate for these problems.

The most common reactions that chronically ill people have to memory and concentration difficulties are self-anger, frustration, and, ultimately, depression.

To cope with your frustration, consider the following suggestions: Even if you falter in your train of thought, or forget what you were going to do next, you can remain calm and possibly retrieve the information you need. You can tell yourself, "I have just misplaced a particular thought. I'll sit still, close my eyes, use the *re-lax* phrase, and the thought may come back." And it will come back some of the time, if you just allow your brain to function without an emotional reaction. If the thought doesn't come back in a few minutes, you'll probably be able to recapture it later. Getting angry at yourself will only further impair your ability to stay focused on the task at hand.

Finding Your Words

One memory problem that is common among people with CFS is difficulty retrieving specific words to convey a thought, complete a sentence, or simply to carry on a conversation. When you can't find the word or concept, a conversation may be halted by your frustrated attempt to retrieve the precise word. To reduce that type of frustration, tell yourself that you don't have to have the exact words; you only need to convey the idea, which can be expressed in other words. Put together simple phrases that will bring you closer and closer to what you wish to express. Eventually the right words will come to you, because they are encoded in your memory. It's also okay to look to your listener for help. He or she may be willing to take some responsibility to help you through a difficult sentence or two—to ask questions that might bring you around to the word or idea you're seeking. Listener involvement will reduce the pressure on you to find the exact word instantaneously, all the time, by yourself.

Make a Behavioral Checklist

It is helpful to identify your areas of memory difficulty (West 1985). Rather than thinking that your memory is thoroughly impaired, you can more productively identify areas of memory success and memory difficulty. List the most common types of memory tasks you do, and note your success or failure for each. Your list doesn't need to be exhaustive—just pick the first 15–25 memory activities that come to mind. Your list will probably include all the most important activities, including

- Remembering a particular person's name

- Locating an item used only occasionally

- Keeping an appointment

- Finishing an errand

- Recalling the details of a conversation

- Knowing your way to a particular place

- Recognizing a face, and associating it with a name

- Remembering a phone number

List each memory activity on the left side of a sheet of lined paper, writing on every other line. On the right-hand side of the page, estimate how often you do remember or complete the listed task. Use percentages to make your estimates. For instance, you may remember the name of a person you meet 50 percent of the time. You may recall the details of a conversation you had yesterday only 30 percent of the time. Don't be discouraged if your memory profile includes many low percentages. This is common among people with CFS. As you review your list, answer these questions (West 1985) to sharpen your daily memory skill:

- In your daily activities, do you jump from one task to the next without taking the time to think about what you're doing in a way that will make it memorable? Many people with CFS are accustomed to rush, rush, rush. Take the time instead to *focus* on what you're doing so that you really experience it: taste your food, savor an emotional interaction or a moment of tenderness. Think about what you want to learn from that moment—what aspect of it you'd like to retain. *Take your time.* The extra time you take will allow you to acquire the information you need. You can only remember information that you acquire in the first place.

- Do mental pictures come to mind easily and aid your memory? Use mental pictures as often as you can.

- Do you forget things when you use mental pictures? Practice improving their accuracy: distinct mental pictures are easier to remember than vague ones.

- Do your memory successes seem to be based on verbal rather than visual techniques? Work towards improving verbal methods, such as rehearsing the words you want to remember.

- Do you forget your doctor's appointment because you thought you'd remember without trying? Next time, make a special effort to remember. Write notes to yourself in a datebook that you carry with you everywhere.

- Do you forget to do errands even if you thought about them repeatedly? Next time, try using visual cues or associations to remind you: Write yourself notes, or tell yourself, for instance, that you'll remember to take your vitamins when you put the water on for your tea.

- Do you mainly remember information that you write down? Use notes more often then.

- Do you write notes to yourself and then lose them? You need to establish a place that you'll always use. A datebook works nicely for many people. You might also want to try a clipboard in your car, or on the refrigerator door.

In general, try to *pattern* your day into a routine in which tasks and activities are scheduled, and things to remember are posted in one specific place.

Other Memory Enhancers

The following suggestions are adapted from the book *Super Memory* by Dr. Douglas Hermann (1992).

- Bad moods, depression, and anxiety will negatively affect your memory. Learn to minimize these mental intrusions (Step 5). If you're depressed or highly agitated, you won't be able to pay attention, or focus your thoughts on something you need to remember. Even if you try to concentrate, you'll have a hard time remembering. Feelings of guilt or excessive worry about minor problems can dominate your thinking and make it almost impossible to recall events you once remembered easily. The slowing down of thinking, often associated with depression, makes it difficult to apply effective memory strategies. You need to recognize when your emotional state has affected your thinking ability, apart from the illness. The stress-control techniques of earlier chapters will help to moderate the negative effects of emotions on your ability to remember.

- Be aware of your memory choices. Focus your attention on retaining particular information, and don't pay much attention to other things. What are the most important things you wish to remember today? Focus in on these using memory aids—stick-on notes, a beeper, an egg timer, or another signaling device. The more selective you are about what you choose to remember, the greater the likelihood that you'll retain the information. Most of the details of your day will be forgotten: this is a normal process of mental filtering, and only partly related to your illness. Allow yourself the right to forget less important things.

- Take mental snapshots. When you lose your train of thought, or forget where you put something, spare yourself frustration and try the following: Sit down, relax a moment, close your eyes, and visualize the situation leading up to the point of memory loss. Re-create the scene as faithfully as possible. Ask yourself questions about it. For instance, if you've lost your car keys, sit down, relax, visualize the last time you remember having them. Continue creating mental snapshots leading you forward in time until you identify the first scene in which you did not have the keys. Shift back and forth between scenes. Visualization aids recall; and it's much faster and more efficient than turning your house upside down, and getting frustrated looking for the keys.

- Use your relaxation techniques before studying, learning, or reading to reduce confusion and improve attention.

- Designate one spot in your home or office to put things that you ordinarily forget to take with you.

- Put cues in visible places: a pill bottle to remind you to go to the doctor, a catalog to remind you to place an order, an empty juice container to remind you of needed grocery items.

- "Sing" the information to be remembered—put the words to a tune and sing them out loud. Because this is such a strange maneuver, you are more likely to remember the content.

You may find some of the following additional suggestions, adopted from Dr. D. G. Cohen, helpful in improving attention and mental alertness.

- Plan low-effort activities (such as reading for pleasure, or writing) that stimulate your interest, and intersperse them throughout your schedule.

- It's important not to become overstimulated in the midst of too much activity going on. Keep distractions to an absolute minimum! Do not, for example, attempt to read with the radio on, or attempt to balance a checkbook while others are in the room talking.

- Watch for signs of increased mental fatigue, and take necessary rest breaks.

- Break down all tasks and activities into incremental steps. Focus only on step one, until it is successfully completed, before moving on to step two.

- Use wall charts, appointment books, calendars, or other tools that will assist you in scheduling and remembering. Use brightly colored markers for emphasis. *Write down everything.* Remember that your goal is memory success— external strategies will improve your chance of accurate recall. Don't be *macho* about it. If success is guaranteed by using a day-book, then use a day-book. Why not?

- Use imagery whenever you can to recall specific information that is difficult to remember. For example, you may recall what you need at the grocery store by forming a mental picture of the meal you intended to prepare. Try reading out loud when you're having trouble focusing on the words. By doing this, you encode the information in three different ways—through seeing it, saying it, and hearing it. This will give you a better chance of assimilating the material and recalling it later on.

All of the above suggestions will help you maximize your cognitive efficiency, and will increase your feelings of control over your illness.

Final Thoughts

Two recent books on CFS have used the terms "curing" and "recovery" in reference to the illness. Although spontaneous recovery certainly occurs, no cure has yet been found. While I remain optimistic that CFS will eventually yield its mysteries to definitive diagnosis, treatment, and cure, I would prefer to use the terms, cope, improve, and function rather than the more incredible word, cure.

Of course, hope is always justified, because many people do improve and function better. In this book, I have presented effective, scientifically based coping strategies. Although these strategies do not eliminate illness issues, they provide a basis for effective, rewarding daily living. As I wrote this book, I began to recognize that, despite my efforts to keep current in the field, I often lose sight of effective coping techniques. I sometimes assume that I practice all the useful methods available to people with CFS. But, in fact, it is all too easy to pursue a daily routine that ignores coping skills that work. At any one moment, it is easier to do what is familiar than what might be most useful to our emotional well-being. And it can be difficult to keep one's mind open and attuned to other people's good ideas. Your knowledge and awareness of whatever positive coping skills are out there will minimize your discouragement and maximize your productivity. I hope that the ideas presented in this book will be a useful adjunct to your effort to function as well as you possibly can.

Appendix A

1994 Case Definition of CFS

Clinically evaluated, unexplained chronic fatigue cases can be separated into either CFS or idiopathic chronic fatigue on the basis of the following criteria:

1. A case of CFS is defined by both a. and b.

   a. Clinically evaluated, unexplained persistent or relapsing chronic fatigue that i) is of new or definite onset (i.e., not lifelong), ii) is not the result of ongoing exertion, iii) is not substantially alleviated by rest, and iv) results in substantial reduction in previous levels of work, study, social, or personal activities.

   b. The concurrent occurrence of four or more of the following symptoms. All of the symptoms must have persisted or recurred during six or more consecutive months of illness and not predated the fatigue. The symptoms are i) self-reported persistent or recurrent impairment in short-term memory or concentration severe enough to cause substantial reduction in previous levels of work, study, social, or personal activities, ii) sore throat, iii) tender neck or axillary lymph nodes, iv) muscle pain, v) multi-joint pain without joint swelling or redness, vi) headaches of a new type, pattern, or severity, vii) unrefreshing sleep, and viii) post-exertional malaise lasting more than 24 hours.

The method used (e.g., use of a predetermined checklist by the investigator or spontaneous reporting by the study participant) to establish the presence of these and any other symptoms should be specified.

2. A case of idiopathic chronic fatigue is defined by clinically evaluated, unexplained chronic fatigue and the failure to meet CFS criteria. The reasons for failing to meet CFS defining criteria should be specified.

Appendix B

Pleasant Events Checklist

This checklist is designed to find out about the things you enjoy, and to give you new ideas about pleasant things to do. The checklist contains a list of events and activities, not all of which will appeal to you (what is pleasant to one person may be torture to another!).

☐ Being in the country

☐ Wearing expensive or formal clothes

☐ Making contributions to religious, charitable, or other groups

☐ Talking about sports

☐ Meeting someone new of the same sex

☐ Taking tests when well-prepared

☐ Going to a rock concert

☐ Playing baseball or softball

☐ Planning trips or vacations

☐ Buying things for myself

☐ Being at the beach

☐ Doing artwork (painting, sculpture, drawing, movie-making, etc.)

☐ Rock climbing or mountaineering

☐ Reading the Scriptures or other sacred works

☐ Playing golf

☐ Re-arranging or redecorating my room or house

☐ Going naked

☐ Going to a sports event

☐ Reading a "How To Do It" book or article

☐ Going to the races (horse, car, boat, etc.)

☐ Reading stories, novels, poems, or plays

☐ Going to a bar, tavern, club, etc.

☐ Going to lectures of hearing speakers

☐ Driving skillfully

☐ Breathing clean air

☐ Thinking up or arranging songs or music

☐ Saying something clearly

☐ Boating (canoeing, kayaking, motorboating, sailing, etc.)

☐ Pleasing my parents

☐ Restoring antiques, refinishing furniture, etc.

☐ Watching TV

☐ Talking to myself

☐ Camping

☐ Working in politics

☐ Working on machines (cars, bikes, motorcycles, tractors, etc.)

☐ Thinking about something good in the future

☐ Playing cards

☐ Completing a difficult task

☐ Laughing

☐ Solving a problem, puzzle, crossword, etc.

☐ Being at weddings, baptisms, confirmations, etc.

☐ Criticizing someone

☐ Shaving

☐ Having lunch with friends or associates

☐ Playing tennis

☐ Taking a shower

☐ Driving long distances

☐ Woodworking, carpentry

☐ Writing stories, novels, plays, or poetry

☐ Being with animals

☐ Riding in an airplane

☐ Exploring (hiking away from known routes, spelunking, etc.)

☐ Having a frank and open conversation

☐ Singing in a group

☐ Thinking about myself or my problems

☐ Working on my job

☐ Going to a party

☐ Going to church functions (socials, classes, bazaars, etc.)

☐ Speaking a foreign language

☐ Going to service, civic, or social club meetings

☐ Going to a business meeting or convention

☐ Being in a sporty or expensive car

☐ Playing a musical instrument

☐ Making snacks

☐ Snow skiing

☐ Being helped

☐ Wearing informal clothes

☐ Combing or brushing my hair

☐ Acting

☐ Taking a nap

☐ Being with friends

☐ Canning, freezing, making preserves, etc.

☐ Driving fast

☐ Solving a personal problem

☐ Being in a city

☐ Taking a bath

☐ Singing to myself

☐ Making food or crafts to sell or give away

☐ Playing pool or billiards

☐ Being with my children or grandchildren

☐ Playing chess or checkers

☐ Doing craft work (pottery, jewelry, leather, beads, weaving, etc.)

☐ Weighing myself

☐ Scratching myself

☐ Putting on make-up, fixing my hair, etc.

☐ Designing or drafting

☐ Visiting people who are sick, shut in, or in trouble

☐ Cheering, rooting

☐ Bowling

☐ Being popular at a gathering

☐ Watching wild animals

☐ Having an original idea

☐ Gardening, landscaping, or doing yard work

☐ Going shopping

☐ Reading essays or technical, academic, or professional literature

☐ Wearing new clothes

☐ Dancing

☐ Sitting in the sun

☐ Riding a motorcycle

☐ Just sitting and thinking

☐ Seeing good things happen to my family or friends

☐ Going to a fair, carnival, circus, zoo, or amusement park

☐ Talking about philosophy or religion

☐ Gambling

☐ Planning or organizing something

☐ Having a drink by myself

☐ Listening to the sounds of nature

☐ Dating, courting, etc.

☐ Having a lively talk

☐ Racing in a car, motorcycle, boat, etc.

☐ Listening to the radio

☐ Having friends come to visit

☐ Playing in a sporting competition

☐ Introducing people who I think would like each other

☐ Giving gifts

☐ Going to school or government meetings, court sessions, etc.

☐ Getting massages or backrubs

☐ Getting letters, cards, or notes

☐ Watching the sky, clouds, or a storm

☐ Going on outings (to the park, a picnic, or a barbecue, etc.)

☐ Playing basketball

☐ Buying something for my family

☐ Photography

☐ Giving a speech or lecture

☐ Reading maps

☐ Gathering natural objects (wild foods or fruit, rocks, driftwood, etc.)

☐ Working on my finances

☐ Wearing clean clothes

☐ Making a major purchase or investment (car, appliance, house, stocks, etc.)

☐ Helping someone

☐ Being in the mountains

☐ Getting a job advancement (being promoted, getting a raise or a better job, being accepted into a better school, etc.)

☐ Hearing jokes

☐ Winning a bet

☐ Talking about my children or grandchildren

☐ Meeting someone new of the opposite sex

☐ Going to a revival meeting or crusade

☐ Talking about my health

☐ Seeing beautiful scenery

☐ Eating good meals

☐ Improving my health (having my teeth fixed, getting new glasses, changing my diet, etc.)

☐ Being downtown

☐ Wrestling or boxing

☐ Hunting or shooting

☐ Playing in a musical group

☐ Hiking

- ☐ Going to a museum or exhibit
- ☐ Writing papers, essays, articles, reports, memos, etc.
- ☐ Doing a job well
- ☐ Having spare time
- ☐ Fishing
- ☐ Loaning something
- ☐ Being noticed as sexually attractive
- ☐ Pleasing employers, teachers, etc.
- ☐ Counseling someone
- ☐ Going to a health club, sauna bath, etc.
- ☐ Having someone give me constructive feedback
- ☐ Learning to do something new
- ☐ Going to a "Drive-in" (Dairy Queen, McDonald's, etc.)
- ☐ Complimenting or praising someone
- ☐ Thinking about people I like
- ☐ Being at a fraternity or sorority
- ☐ Being with my parents
- ☐ Horseback riding
- ☐ Protesting social, political, or environmental conditions
- ☐ Talking on the telephone
- ☐ Having daydreams
- ☐ Kicking leaves, sand, pebbles, etc.
- ☐ Playing lawn sports (badminton, croquet, shuffleboard, horse-shoes, etc.)
- ☐ Going to school reunions, alumni meetings, etc.
- ☐ Seeing famous people
- ☐ Going to the movies
- ☐ Kissing
- ☐ Being alone

- ☐ Budgeting my time
- ☐ Cooking meals
- ☐ Being praised by people I admire
- ☐ Outwitting a "superior"
- ☐ Feeling the presence of the Lord in my life
- ☐ Doing a project in my own way
- ☐ Doing odd jobs around the house
- ☐ Having a good cry
- ☐ Being at a family reunion or get-together
- ☐ Giving a party or get-together
- ☐ Washing my hair
- ☐ Coaching someone
- ☐ Going to a restaurant
- ☐ Seeing or smelling a flower or plant
- ☐ Being invited out
- ☐ Receiving honors (civic, military, etc.)
- ☐ Using cologne, perfume, or aftershave
- ☐ Having someone agree with me
- ☐ Reminiscing, talking about old times
- ☐ Getting up early in the morning
- ☐ Having peace and quiet
- ☐ Doing experiments or other scientific work
- ☐ Visiting friends
- ☐ Writing in a diary
- ☐ Playing football
- ☐ Being counseled
- ☐ Saying prayers
- ☐ Giving massages or backrubs

- [ ] Hitchhiking
- [ ] Meditating or doing yoga
- [ ] Doing favors for people
- [ ] Talking with people on the job or in class
- [ ] Being relaxed
- [ ] Being asked for my help or advice
- [ ] Thinking about other people's problems
- [ ] Playing board games (Monopoly, Scrabble, etc.)
- [ ] Sleeping soundly at night
- [ ] Doing heavy outdoor work (cutting or chopping wood, clearing land, farm work, etc.)
- [ ] Reading the newspaper
- [ ] Snowmobiling or dune-buggy riding
- [ ] Being in a body-awareness, sensitivity, encounter, therapy, or "rap" group
- [ ] Dreaming at night
- [ ] Playing ping pong
- [ ] Brushing my teeth
- [ ] Swimming
- [ ] Running, jogging, or doing gymnastic, fitness, or field exercises
- [ ] Walking barefoot
- [ ] Playing frisbee or catch
- [ ] Doing housework or laundry; cleaning things
- [ ] Being with my roommate
- [ ] Listening to music
- [ ] Arguing
- [ ] Knitting, crocheting, embroidery, or fancy needlework
- [ ] Petting, necking

☐ Amusing people

☐ Talking about sex

☐ Having houseguests

☐ Being with someone I love

☐ Reading magazines

☐ Sleeping late

☐ Starting a new project

☐ Being stubborn

☐ Having sex

☐ Having other sexual satisfactions

☐ Going to the library

☐ Playing soccer, rugby, hockey, lacrosse, etc.

☐ Preparing a new or special food

☐ Birdwatching

☐ Watching people

☐ Building or watching a fire

☐ Winning an argument

☐ Selling or trading something

☐ Finishing a project or task

☐ Confessing or apologizing

☐ Repairing things

☐ Working with others as a team

☐ Bicycling

☐ Telling people what to do

☐ Being with happy people

☐ Playing party games

☐ Writing letters, cards, or notes

☐ Talking about politics or public affairs

☐ Asking for help or advice

☐ Going to banquets, luncheons, potlucks, etc.

☐ Talking about my hobby or special interest

☐ Watching attractive women or men

☐ Smiling at people

☐ Playing in sand, a stream, the grass, etc.

☐ Talking about other people

☐ Being with my husband or wife

☐ Having people show interest in what I have said

☐ Going on field trips, nature walks, etc.

☐ Expressing my love to someone

☐ Caring for houseplants

☐ Having coffee, tea, a coke, etc., with friends

☐ Taking a walk

☐ Collecting things

☐ Playing handball, paddleball, squash, etc.

☐ Sewing

☐ Remembering a departed friend or loved one, visiting the cemetery

☐ Doing things with children

☐ Beachcombing

☐ Being complimented or told I have done well

☐ Being told I am loved

☐ Eating snacks

☐ Staying up late

☐ Having family members or friends do something that makes me proud of them

☐ Being with my children

☐ Going to auctions, garage sales, etc.

☐ Thinking about an interesting question

☐ Doing volunteer work; working on community service projects

☐ Water skiing, surfing, scuba diving

☐ Receiving money

☐ Defending or protecting someone; stopping fraud or abuse

☐ Hearing a good sermon

☐ Picking up a hitchhiker

☐ Winning a competition

☐ Making a new friend

☐ Talking about my job or school

☐ Reading cartoons, comic strips, or comic books

☐ Borrowing something

☐ Traveling with a group

☐ Seeing old friends

☐ Teaching someone

☐ Using my strength

☐ Traveling

☐ Going to office parties or departmental get-togethers

☐ Attending a concert, opera, or ballet

☐ Playing with pets

☐ Going to a play

☐ Looking at the stars or moon

☐ Being coached

Adapted from MacPhillamy and Lewinsohn (1982).

Appendix C

Coping Strategies Gathered From Around the World

- "Stop immediately when fatigued."
- "Nap or rest 3–4 hours even on a good day."
- "Work a little, rest a little, etc."
- "When I become very tired, I've learned I need to give in to it."
- "Have a comfortable place to rest outside and enjoy nature."
- "Rest when you're not well, even if people give you a hard time."
- "Avoid stress."
- "Refuse to argue about things—it drains energy."
- "Start Christmas shopping in March."
- "Give other family members more responsibilities."
- "Learn to build a new life."

- "Read uplifting, spiritual books, watch funny TV shows."
- "Phone others who are ill, and try to help them know they're not alone."
- "Conserve energy for important things so as to not miss out on life."
- "When making plans, always try to take your variable health into consideration."
- "Weigh if an activity or social event is worth the suffering afterwards."
- "Remember always that relationships get top priority when energy is low."
- "Don't waste energy explaining your condition to skeptics."
- "Try to have the peace of mind that you can go through life without everyone understanding."
- "Avoid people who stress you."
- "Find rewarding things you can do to bolster your self-image/esteem and sense of control."
- "Accept, trust, and love yourself, no matter what."
- "Find escapes that work for you (movies, books, special friends, etc.)."
- "Humor, humor, and more humor."
- "Avoid contact with people who have attitudes of 'you could get better if you really . . . ,' including your family."
- "Make lists noting one or two priority activities a day. If you do them, you'll feel better and things aren't such a mess."
- "Try to remember that bad days will pass, and you will feel better for some (unknown) period of time."
- "Change your priorities."
- "Don't waste time worrying about what could have been."
- "Simplify, lower, limit goals."
- "What is, is enough."

- "Be in the moment—it contains all of life."
- "Ask what is the lesson? What is the purpose?"
- "Never stop believing in yourself."
- "Use phone networking with other people with CFS for support."
- "Allow yourself to be good to yourself."
- "Try to involve yourself in helping others."
- "Unload emotionally or physically draining friendships and relationships."
- "Get a H.U.D. apartment."
- "Healthy lifestyle, strict diet."
- "Live with animals."
- "Pray to God."
- "Optimize use of appliances."
- "Use stick-on notes in your purse—each time I open my purse, I'm reminded of what I need to do."
- "Use a speaker phone if your arms are weak."
- "If you have left a message for someone to return your call, leave that person's name circled on a pad, with a note of what you'd called about, near your phone."
- "Get washed and dressed and go out every day, even if just to drive to the video store."
- "Feel the pain rather than take pills or distract yourself."
- "Pace yourself—engage in fun, pleasurable activities as much as possible."
- "Keep busy by learning new things—try correspondence school."
- "Yoga, sunshine, diet, sleep, and no stress."
- "Take charge—doctors give advice, but you make the decisions."

- "When spent, use a wheelchair to conserve strength."
- "Evoke good memories, triumphs, and laughter."
- "Use lightweight tools and cooking utensils."
- "Diet, nutrition, relaxation tapes."
- "Practice optimism (some call this denial)."
- "Break all tasks into pieces and tackle only one at a time. Drop out for periods of time (let yourself crash)."
- "Let the house be dirty, order a pizza, or use freezer dinners."
- "Hire a cleaning lady."
- "Get groceries delivered."
- "Accept that you have an illness that prevents you from being your once-energetic self."
- "Stop feeling guilty for what you can't do, and mentally or verbally praise yourself for what you do get done."
- "Don't make a fulfilling life contingent upon being well."
- "Dream about a cure/treatment."
- "Keep a sense of humor."
- "Find the small joys of life."
- "Do something every day—dishes one day, dust one day, wash clothes another, etc."
- "Exercise (if you can)."
- "Find the level of exercise you can tolerate, and don't exceed it."
- "No unnecessary exercise."
- "Mild exercise—slow swimming."
- "Listen to your body."
- "Go on-line and learn everything you can about your illness."
- "Don't forget to say your prayers."
- "Ask for help when you need it."

- "Say no."
- "Write—often in prayer form."
- "Be smart, if not smarter than your doctor."
- "Try not to compare yourself to healthy friends."
- "Use a scooter, a disabled parking permit, and do a lot by phone."
- "Always look forward to tomorrow."
- "Do crossword puzzles to keep your mind reasonably sharp."
- "Shop early—grocery and drug store—no lines."
- "Firmly believe that you have value as a human being, even though you're ill."
- "Psychotherapy."
- "Acknowledge the illness, quit pretending."
- "Go to a support group—they give and receive help; donate money for research."
- "Develop a personal physical therapy program to help pain (regular physical therapy programs can make it worse)."
- "Do get things done during the time when you have more energy, even if they aren't required until later (fixing lunch, dinner, etc)."
- "Simplify your life to whatever degree is possible."
- "Try to keep active just short of relapse."
- "Don't discuss the illness with anyone but your doctor, other people with CFS, or your spouse. Former co-workers, friends just don't believe you have an illness. Trying to explain CFS is just frustrating."
- "Let go of anal-retentive, perfectionist tendencies."
- "Accept that you're okay anyway, even if you can't drive or listen or whatever. You're okay."
- "Don't give up all your aspirations and interests."

- "Avoid stores, driving, or using buses."
- "Saturate your life with beautiful people and things; eliminate critical, judgmental people and their twisted thinking."
- "Give books, videos, etc. along with info on CFS to your doctor and any other doctor who will read—also congresspersons, etc."
- "Always plan to do fun things, even if you need to cancel sometimes."
- "Use medications that help without guilt."
- "Live one day at a time."
- "Just scream sometimes."
- "Develop acceptance of your condition, limitations, and their effect on your life—not in terms of defeat, but in terms of having a different way of living and functioning as best you can within these differences."
- "Accept the reality of your mostly unpredictable level of function, with humor, and recognize your desire that you be other than what you are whenever it pops up."
- "Keep informed about CFS and consider your options."
- "At the first sign of relapse, rest until your symptoms abate."
- "Use self-hypnosis to beat the pains in joints and muscles."

Adapted from a list compiled by Marjorie J. McKenzie II, M.A., from a study of long-term CFS.

To order the audiocassette tape with relaxation and stress reduction techniques and coping messages for chronic fatigue syndrome, please send a check or money order for $9.00 to Fred Friedberg, Ph.D., P.O. Box 456, Kent, CT 06757. You will receive the tape within two weeks of receipt of your order.

Bibliography

Abbey, S.E., & Garfinkel, P.E. 1991. "Neurasthenia and Chronic Fatigue Syndrome: The Role of Culture in the Making of a Diagnosis." *American Journal of Psychiatry* 148:1638-1646.

Berk, L.S. et al. 1989. "Neuroendocrine and Stress Hormone Changes During Mirthful Laughter." *American Journal of Medical Sciences* 298:390-396.

Brown, W.A. et al. 1993. "Endocrine Correlates of Sadness and Elation." *Psychosomatic Medicine,* 55:458-467.

Butler, S., Chalder, T., Ron, M., & Wessely, S. 1990. "Cognitive Behaviour Therapy in Chronic Fatigue Syndrome." *Journal of Neurology Neurosurgery and Psychiatry* 54; 305:147-152.

Cousins, N. 1989. *Head First: The Biology of Hope.* New York: E.P. Dutton.

Dechene, L. 1993. "Chronic Fatigue Syndrome. Influence of Histamine, Hormones and Electrolytes." *Medical Hypotheses,* 40:55-60.

DeLuca, J., Johnson, S.K., & Natelson, B.H. 1993. "Information Processing Efficiency in Chronic Fatigue Syndrome and Multiple Sclerosis." *Archives of Neurology* 50:301-304.

Demitrack, M.A., et al. 1991. "Evidence for the Impaired Activation of the Hypothalamic-pituitary-adrenal Axis in Patients with Chronic Fatigue Syndrome." *Journal of Clinical Endocrinology and Metabolism* 73: 1-11.

Denz-Penhey, H., & Murdoch, J.C. 1993. "Service Delivery for People with Chronic Fatigue Syndrome: A Pilot Action Research Study." *Family Practice* 10:14-18.

Ellis, A. 1973. *A Guide to Rational Living.* North Hollywood: Wilshire Book Company.

Fennel, P.A. In press. "Chronic Fatigue Syndrome: Sociocultural Influences and Trauma: Clinical Considerations." *Journal of Chronic Fatigue Syndrome.*

Friedberg, F., & Krupp, L.B. 1994. "A Comparison of Cognitive Behavioral Treatment for Chronic Fatigue Syndrome and Primary Depression." *Clinical Infectious Diseases*: 18 (Suppl. 1), S105-S110.

Friedberg, F., McKenzie, M., Dechene, L., & Fontanetta, R. 1994. "Symptom Patterns and Illness Progression in Long-term Chronic Fatigue Syndrome." Paper presented at the American Association for Chronic Fatigue Syndrome conference in Ft. Lauderdale, Florida.

Fukuda, K., et al. 1994. "Chronic Fatigue Syndrome: A Comprehensive Approach to its Definition and Study." *Annals of Internal Medicine* 121:953-959.

Goodman, J. 1988. "Managing Humor." *Laughing Matters* 5:24-25.

Gunn, W.J., Connell, D.B., & Randall, B. 1993. "Epidemiology of Chronic Fatigue Syndrome: The Centers-for-Disease-Control Study." In B.R. Bock & J. Whelan (Eds.), *Chronic Fatigue Syndrome*, pp. 83-101. New York: John Wiley & Sons.

Grissom Productions, Inc. 1994. Tapes of the 1994 meeting of the American Association for Chronic Fatigue Syndrome. 904 South 22nd Street, Arlington, VA 22202; tel. 1-800-484-7447.

Hermann, D. 1992. *Supermemory.* Avenul, New Jersey: Outlet Book Company.

Hickie, I., Wakefield, D., Boughton, C.R., & Owyer, J. 1993. "A Double Blind, Placebo-controlled Trial of Intraverons Immunoglobulin in Patients with Chronic Fatigue Syndrome." *American Journal of Medicine* 94:197-203.

Holmes, G.P., et al. 1988. "Chronic Fatigue Syndrome: A Working Case Definition." *Annals of Internal Medicine* 108:387-389.

Jason, L.A. 1993. "Chronic Fatigue Syndrome: New Hope from Psychneuroimmunology and Community Psychology." *The Journal of Primary Prevention* 14:51-71.

Keim, K. 1994. "Patient's Perspective: Improve Your Sleep; Feel Better." *The CFIDS Chronicle* 20-21 (Winter).

Klein, A. 1989. *The Healing Power of Humor*. Los Angeles, Jeremy P. Tarcher.

Krupp, L.B., Sliwinski, M., Masur, D.M., Friedberg, F., & Coyle, P.K. 1994. "Cognitive Functioning and Depression in Patients with Chronic Fatigue Syndrome and Multiple Schlerosis." *Archives of Neurology* 57:705-710.

Lapp, C. 1994. "Chronic Fatigue Syndrome." Presentation given to the Connecticut CFIDS Association, Inc.

Lewis, G., & Wessely, S. 1992. "The Epidemiology of Fatigue: More Questions Than Answers." *Journal of Epidemiology and Community Health* 46:92-97.

Lutgendorf, S. et al. In press. "Physical Symptoms of Chronic Fatigue Syndrome Are Exacerbated by the Stress of Hurricane Andrew." *Psychosomatic Medicine.*

MacPhillamy, D.J., & Lewinsohn, D.M. 1982. "The Pleasant Events Schedule: Studies on Reliability, Validity, and Scale Construction." *Journal of Consulting and Clinical Psychology* 50:363-380.

Morgan, A.E. 1942. *The Small Community*. Yellow Springs, Ohio: Community Service, Inc.

Pennebaker, J., Kiecolt-Glaser, J.K., & Glaser, R. 1988. "Disclosure of Traumas and Immune Function: Health Implications for Psychotherapy." *Journal of Consulting and Clinical Psychology* 56:239-245.

Ray, C. 1992. "Positive and Negative Social Support in a Chronic Illness." *Psychological Reports* 71:977-978.

Rogers, S. 1986. *The E.I. Syndrome. An Rx for Environmental Illness.* Syracuse, NY: Prestige.

Schluederberg, A., et al. 1992. "Chronic Fatigue Syndrome Research: Definition and Medical Outcome Assessment." *Annals of Internal Medicine* 117:325-331.

Schwartz, R.B., et al. 1994. "Detection of Intracranial Abnormalities in Patients with Chronic Fatigue Syndrome: Comparison of MR Imaging and SPECT." *American Journal of Roentgenology* 162:935-951.

Siegel, B. 1986. *Love, Medicine and Miracles*. New York: Harper & Row.

Spacapan, S., & Oskamp, S. (Eds.). 1992. *Helping and Being Helped.* Newburg Park, CA: Sage.

Stone, A.A., et al. 1994. "Fatigue and Mood in Chronic Fatigue Syndrome Patients: Results of a Momentous Assessment Protocol Examining Fatigue and Mood Levels and Diurnal Patterns." *Annals of Behavioral Medicine* 16:228-234.

Strayer, D.R., et al. 1994. "A Controlled Clinical Trial With a Specifically Configured RNA Drug, Poly(I)-Poly($C_{12}U$), in Chronic Fatigue Syndrome." *Clinical Infectious Diseases,* 18:S88-S95.

Tubesing, N.L., & Tubesing, D.A. 1983. "Structural Exercises in Stress Management." Duluth, MN: Whole Person Press.

Ware, N.C. 1993. "Society, Mind and Body in Chronic Fatigue Syndrome: An Anthropological View." In G.R. Boch & J. Whelan (Eds.), *Chronic fatigue syndrome,* pp. 62-81. New York: John Wiley.

Weekes, C. 1969. *Hope and Help for Your Nerves.* New York: Hawthorn Books.

West, R. 1985. *Memory Fitness Over 40.* Gainsville, FL: Triad Publishing.

Wilson, A., et al. 1994. "Longitudinal Study of Outcome of Chronic Fatigue Syndrome." *British Medical Journal* 308:756-759.

Wood, C., Magnello, M., & Sharpe, M. 1992. "Fluctuations in Perceived Energy and Mood Among Patients with Chronic Fatigue Syndrome." *Journal of the Royal Society of Medicine* 85:195-198.

Other New Harbinger Self-Help Titles

Flying Without Fear, $12.95
Kid Cooperation: How to Stop Yelling, Nagging & Pleading and Get Kids to Cooperate, $12.95
The Stop Smoking Workbook: Your Guide to Healthy Quitting, $17.95
Conquering Carpal Tunnel Syndrome and Other Repetitive Strain Injuries, $17.95
The Tao of Conversation, $12.95
Wellness at Work: Building Resilience for Job Stress, $14.95
What Your Doctor Can't Tell You About Cosmetic Surgery, $13.95
An End of Panic: Breakthrough Techniques for Overcoming Panic Disorder, $17.95
On the Clients Path: A Manual for the Practice of Solution-Focused Therapy, $39.95
Living Without Procrastination: How to Stop Postponing Your Life, $12.95
Goodbye Mother, Hello Woman: Reweaving the Daughter Mother Relationship, $14.95
Letting Go of Anger: The 10 Most Common Anger Styles and What to Do About Them, $12.95
Messages: The Communication Skills Workbook, Second Edition, $13.95
Coping With Chronic Fatigue Syndrome: Nine Things You Can Do, $12.95
The Anxiety & Phobia Workbook, Second Edition, $15.95
Thueson's Guide to Over-The Counter Drugs, $13.95
Natural Women's Health: A Guide to Healthy Living for Women of Any Age, $13.95
I'd Rather Be Married: Finding Your Future Spouse, $13.95
The Relaxation & Stress Reduction Workbook, Fourth Edition, $17.95
Living Without Depression & Manic Depression: A Workbook for Maintaining Mood Stability, $17.95
Belonging: A Guide to Overcoming Loneliness, $13.95
Coping With Schizophrenia: A Guide For Families, $13.95
Visualization for Change, Second Edition, $13.95
Postpartum Survival Guide, $13.95
Angry All The Time: An Emergency Guide to Anger Control, $12.95
Couple Skills: Making Your Relationship Work, $13.95
Handbook of Clinical Psychopharmacology for Therapists, $39.95
The Warrior's Journey Home: Healing Men, Healing the Planet, $13.95
Weight Loss Through Persistence, $13.95
Post-Traumatic Stress Disorder: A Complete Treatment Guide, $39.95
Stepfamily Realities: How to Overcome Difficulties and Have a Happy Family, $13.95
Leaving the Fold: A Guide for Former Fundamentalists and Others Leaving Their Religion, $13.95
Father-Son Healing: An Adult Son's Guide, $12.95
The Chemotherapy Survival Guide, $11.95
Your Family/Your Self: How to Analyze Your Family System, $12.95
Being a Man: A Guide to the New Masculinity, $12.95
The Deadly Diet, Second Edition: Recovering from Anorexia & Bulimia, $13.95
Last Touch: Preparing for a Parent's Death, $11.95
Consuming Passions: Help for Compulsive Shoppers, $11.95
Self-Esteem, Second Edition, $13.95
I Can't Get Over It, A Handbook for Trauma Survivors, $13.95
Concerned Intervention, When Your Loved One Won't Quit Alcohol or Drugs, $11.95
Dying of Embarrassment: Help for Social Anxiety and Social Phobia, $12.95
The Depression Workbook: Living With Depression and Manic Depression, $14.95
The Marriage Bed: Renewing Love, Friendship, Trust, and Romance, $11.95
Focal Group Psychotherapy: For Mental Health Professionals, $44.95
Hot Water Therapy: Save Your Back, Neck & Shoulders in 10 Minutes a Day $11.95
Prisoners of Belief: Exposing & Changing Beliefs that Control Your Life, $10.95
Be Sick Well: A Healthy Approach to Chronic Illness, $11.95
Men & Grief: A Guide for Men Surviving the Death of a Loved One., $12.95
When the Bough Breaks: A Helping Guide for Parents of Sexually Abused Childern, $11.95
Love Addiction: A Guide to Emotional Independence, $12.95
When Once Is Not Enough: Help for Obsessive Compulsives, $13.95
The New Three Minute Meditator, $12.95
Getting to Sleep, $12.95
Beyond Grief: A Guide for Recovering from the Death of a Loved One, $13.95
Leader's Guide to the Relaxation & Stress Reduction Workbook, Fourth Edition, $19.95
The Divorce Book, $11.95
Hypnosis for Change: A Manual of Proven Techniques, 2nd Edition, $13.95
The Chronic Pain Control Workbook, $14.95
When Anger Hurts, $13.95
Free of the Shadows: Recovering from Sexual Violence, $12.95
Lifetime Weight Control, $11.95
Love and Renewal: A Couple's Guide to Commitment, $13.95

Call **toll free, 1-800-748-6273**, to order. Have your Visa or Mastercard number ready. Or send a check for the titles you want to New Harbinger Publications, Inc., 5674 Shattuck Avenue, Oakland, CA 94609. Include $3.80 for the first book and 75¢ for each additional book, to cover shipping and handling. (California residents please include appropriate sales tax.) Allow four to six weeks for delivery.

Prices subject to change without notice.